Remember Joan

An Alzheimer's Story

Candace Minor Comstock

DEDICATION

For my mother and all her wisdom

CONTENTS

ACKNOWLEDGMENTS

First and foremost, I must thank my husband, Steve. Your love and support has forever enriched my life.

Thank you, Bonnie and Lee, for being such great kids. I love you both beyond words.

Thanks to Scott for traveling this journey by my side, and thanks to Lea Anne for listening all these years.

Heartfelt thanks to all the friends and family for the wonderful memories expressed in this work.

My appreciation also goes out to Olga who provided brilliant editing services and creative direction.

Chapter 1   The Wedding

You would have loved the wedding, Mom. We would have cherished your presence. Other than the short tribute I gave to you and the murmurings that must have gone on well hidden from my ears, it was a fun wedding that showed no signs of following a funeral. Everyone grabbed my hand that night and said, "Your daughter is beautiful. This wedding is fabulous." No one on that night held my hand and said, "I'm sorry to hear about your mother. She was such a great lady."

We had the wedding at the house, Mom. I know you don't remember much about our recent home purchase. Steve and I bought a charming twenty-five-year-old Tudor in need of cosmetic updating, a match for us indeed. We made the move to become close to Steve's office, and my transfer to a public school in the area was not a problem. The kids were both away in college, so the community and home of their childhood held fewer ties. The new location was only five miles farther from you than our old house, though in a different direction. But you never managed to drive yourself to our new place. I picked you up often to show you our efforts at home improvement. We still made it a point to get you over for many Sunday dinners. Unfortunately, Mom, your days were passing by in an ever-increasing fog of confusion.

One late afternoon about a year after our relocation, when Steve and I were enjoying some beers after a grueling day of laying bricks for our new patio, we mentioned how perfect this yard would be for a wedding. There were no plans for the kids to get married at that time, not even serious relationships on the go for either of them. It was just a casual, truthful comment. We were relaxing on the deck that overlooked the woods. Everything was so green and peaceful. We looked back at the house and the brick patio that was forming and talked about how pretty white lights in the trees and white covered tables on the bricks would be. The wedding vows could take place where we sat, on the lower deck that shoots out into the lush foliage. Gorgeous. We were just dreaming out loud, as we always do. But like so many other conversations of dreams we engage in, this one also came true.

Mom, you know how hard Steve and I work on home improvement projects and how we like to do it all ourselves. The backyard transformation was no different. There was a stretch of dirt and bits of suffering grass between the house and the steep hill that descended into the wooded valley. Arranging 5000 bricks in the long and narrow yard in a design reminiscent of a Charleston alleyway was our vision.

First, a truckload of dirt was delivered to the house. Once we leveled the yard, the crushed gravel truckload was delivered. Then, the gravel and bricks were laid in small sections. I gathered and delivered the materials to Steve who was on all fours doing the real job of it. Finally, more crushed gravel was swept into the cracks over and over again. You saw the final result the last time you were here for Bonnie's college graduation celebration cookout, but you didn't say a word. Although, I knew just what you would have said if you could. "Candy, you and Steve are such a good team. The work you did is just unbelievable. Your patio is simply beautiful!"

Steve and I are a good team. We are constantly amazed and appreciative of the good fortune bestowed upon us throughout our marriage. Often, when we are experiencing a moment of sappy, heart-warming love for each other, my head breaks into that song Maria and Captain von Trapp sang to each other in *The Sound of Music.* "Nothing comes from nothing/Nothing ever could/Somewhere in my wicked childhood/I must have done something good." I have this habit of silently singing song lyrics that connect to marked moments in my life, a sort of unsophisticated, amateur psychology or philosophy.

Anyway Mom, the news of an upcoming wedding came right after the patio was completed, right when Steve and I were contemplating what our next home project would be. That's about the time Steve got the phone call early in February. Bonnie's boyfriend, Joe, did the old fashioned tradition of asking the father for his daughter's hand in marriage. Steve gave it and added a modern tradition of telling his future son in law that he had to call Bonnie's mother and ask her too! That was just like Steve to want me to experience something unique and wonderful along with him. We were happy to welcome Joe to the family. Joe was the first boyfriend Bonnie brought home to meet us that before five minutes were up I didn't say to myself, "He's not the one."

I thought that four times before. That's how many boyfriends Bonnie had brought home from college.

That's also how many times Bonnie changed her major while attending university. In fact, the changes in boyfriends and majors coincided. I believe the brainy guy went with her chemistry major, the lady's man with her math major, the cop with her psychology major, and the bartender went with her art major. She ultimately decided on mass communications and Joe.

When she brought Joe home the first time, I noticed some really good things. He paid attention to the little brother, Lee. He was interested in what classes Lee was taking in college, what music he liked, what games he played. He hung out with Lee, and Bonnie didn't mind.

The day we went to Dad's house for a visit and a canoe ride on the lake, I was sold on Joe. The hike down to the lake from Dad's house is short but practically vertical. It's really a variation of a cliff. Steve begins the journey each time by staring at all the paraphernalia that has to make it down to the canoe that is waiting at the water's edge at the bottom of the hill-cliff. He has a dolly and must plan out the proper configuration of the incredibly heavy battery, life jackets, fishing poles, tackle boxes, and cooler onto the dolly to reach the canoe in one trip, the goal. While he was organizing it all in his mind, Joe carried the thirty-five pound battery down the hill-cliff and was already on his way back up. Wow, now Steve, Lee, Bonnie, and Joe could easily carry everything that was left to the boat in one trip, smiling all the way. When they reached the bottom, Joe for the second time, Bonnie had something to say. "I wish I remembered to get one of those wine coolers Mom brought with us."

Well, Joe was back up the hill-cliff to fulfill her wish, and I was on the deck grinning and amazed. I was very impressed. It takes most people a while to recover after one trip up the hill-cliff, and Joe's prancing up for the second time in fifteen minutes because Bonnie is thirsty for a margarita wine cooler. Did I tell you he's an eagle scout and a black belt? You met him, Mom. I know you don't remember, but you smiled at him.

With an engagement in place, the wedding plans began. Steve and I wondered how Bonnie and Joe would feel about the idea of a wedding at our home. We knew it would be their decision, and we would go along with any location the bride and groom chose, but we hoped they would like our idea. Joe loved it immediately, and Bonnie had to give it some time and serious thought. I quickly noticed how they would balance each other.

It was decided that the idea could work. Bonnie and I were excited about making plans. She wanted to include you so badly. We told you the news, and you appeared pleased. It was a sad ingredient, your absence in the planning. After all, Mom, you taught me how to throw a great party, making guests feel at home. You were so creative and talented when it came to entertaining. You were at your best celebrating in the company of others. Bonnie and I always pictured you kicking up your heels at her wedding. It was a grim reality for Bonnie, the two of you being so close. Remember when she was little? You used to say you needed your Bonnie fix. From the beginning, you guys enjoyed a special relationship. I know how much joy she brought to your life at a time when you were alone. For Bonnie, a weekend with Grandma meant lunches at fancy downtown restaurants, trips to museums, zoos, parks, anywhere that you could add culture and beauty into her life. You greatly influenced her spirit, and I thank you so much for that,

Mom. It broke my heart you couldn't share this joyful experience with us.

We had six months to create an enchanting wedding set to occur in the evening of the first weekend in October. Bonnie and Joe's engagement was rather short as had been their courtship. But remember, Mom, I did the same thing when I met Steve. Bonnie bought a wedding planner book, and we wrote down the lists of things to do. I recalled how nicely everything went for my wedding, how you and I avoided anxiety and useless tizzies. Luckily, Bonnie continued with our tradition of composure. I researched caterers, and she looked for a photographer.

About that time, Steve came home from work and told me about this great catered lunch his office had provided. He raved about the grilled vegetables. We checked out the company's menus on line, booked a tasting, loved the food, and reserved the caterer. They even took care of the tables and chairs, tablecloths and linen napkins, dishes, glassware, and cutlery. Bonnie loved the name of the caterer, Hugs and Quiches. Bonnie talked to a friend who was recently married about her choice in a wedding photographer. His work was displayed in the college town restaurant where Bonnie waited tables, and she had always admired the photography. After a phone call, he was booked. It was painless so far.

As far as preparing the house for the wedding, Steve and I knew what our next project would be, the outdated, empty basement. That was to be the location for the DJ and dancing. Paint on the old wall paneling and new ceiling tiles were in order. Lea Anne said she'd come over to help me hang white lights behind sheer curtains to make the basement look as good as any reception hall around.

Steve worked on outdoor lights. He traced all the branches along the dogwood tree with the little white lights. Bonnie wanted lights to loop back and forth from the house to the woods, creating a canopy over the brick patio. Of course, Steve figured out how to comply using cables and pulleys. It was like a million tiny stars glittering overhead, anchored by the house and the poplars.

Bonnie and I made the invitations ourselves. We were trying to come up with ways to cut back on expenses. On the Internet we found this recycled paper with embedded fern leaves. We were trying to begin a theme, and the nature, woodsy theme made sense with our outdoor, woodsy setting. So we spent a day printing, cutting, gluing, and assembling the invitations. We sure needed your calligraphy talents, Mom.

We ordered a three tiered chocolate and vanilla wedding cake covered in white and cream frosting roses at the local grocery bakery. A friend of mine recommended a DJ, and Bonnie and Joe came over one night for pizza and conversation about music details. I talked to the orchestra teacher at school, and she agreed to come and play with her quartet before the ceremony and during the procession. The plans were moving forward, but I slowed down telling you everything about the excitement after a while. You usually just looked at me with that blank expression.

When it came time for the dress, like most brides, Bonnie wanted to fall in love. Mom, I remembered the two of us searching together until we found my perfect dress. Bonnie and I began our search one early summer weekend. The first day helped her narrow down her likes and dislikes. You know, the neck of this one was right, and the skirt of that one was right. Most looked gorgeous on her, but we didn't find "the one." The second day we began to see the same dresses. We were hungry for lunch, a little disheartened, and about to leave this shop when the sales clerk stopped us. She mentioned the dress in the window which we had overlooked. She sure had paid attention to our comments entering and leaving the dressing room. The dress was everything Bonnie had been looking for. It was strapless, antique white, adorned with lace and appliqués, entwined with sequins and beads. The neck was sweetheart cut, the skirt A-line, and the train was the right length. It was beautiful and incorporated all the things she had been drawn to. When she stepped into the gown, we knew. Accessorizing with a simple veil, a jeweled hair comb, and ballerina slippers finished her off. Elegant and enchanting, that was our Bonnie.

I found my dress at Dillard's on the clearance rack. My shopping style was passed down directly from you, Mom. Walk quickly to the back of the store in search of red clearance signs. It was the first dress I tried on, and it was perfect. I asked the clerk to hold the dress, and I spent a few more hours looking at other shops just to make sure. Of course, I went back to purchase the original bargain gown. I refused to look at the mother of the bride dresses in pastel colors with matching jackets. My dress was a tan colored, sleeveless, low backed, beaded to the floor beauty. You would have approved.

Bonnie wanted her bridesmaids to wear any style dress they fancied. I liked that idea. She chose a deep red for the color, and all the girls selected a style that suited their figures. The groomsmen were going to wear black suits, which most of them owned. I found the same deep red color necktie at a Ties Are Us type website to complete the look. Bonnie and Joe were being very practical minded.

And get this, we ordered tons of deep red and white spray roses and Queen Anne's lace to be delivered to the house the day before the wedding. That way the girls could design their own bouquets and decorate our yard with the extra flowers on the day of the wedding. Some of the girls were planning on spending the night at the house on the wedding eve to help out on the wedding day.

Best yet, Mom, guess who we asked to marry Bonnie and Joe? Your Scotty! Remember when Scott was an eighteen-year-old hippie and sent away the application to be an ordained minister with Life Universal Church? Well, the demand for secular officiates is on the rise today, Mom, and your son has been quite busy marrying folks. I thought the decision was a beautiful touch, and Bonnie and Joe thought so too. Your other son, Mark, was also on the itinerary. We asked him to play the guitar, and together with Debbie, sing "The Wedding Song," the same rendition that Mark and Debbie performed at Steve's and my wedding.

All the planning leading up to the big day went very smoothly. The week before was predictably crazy busy, but I've heard that's just the way it is no matter how organized a person happens to be. Steve took the whole week off from work, and I had two days to join him. Joe's parents came into town, and after we introduced ourselves and shared words of affection and admiration for each other's children, we handed them brooms and rakes. They had no objections to jumping in to help make everything party ready. Last minute communications with the hotels that were putting up our out of town guests, the transportation arrangements, rehearsal dinner reservations, the caterer, the photographer, the DJ, the quartet, and the officiate all were in order and crossed off the list.

With the wedding set for six o'clock, rain was the only factor that could damage the plans. We did have a tent on reserve just in case. Thankfully, the weather cooperated. It was hotter than usual for October, some humidity in the air, not a bright sunny day, but slightly hazy. The photographer said that kind of lighting was perfect for photographing people. Mom, I would have loved a picture of the three of us, Bonnie, me, and you.

That slightly hazy day began with running out to the nursery and the party store first thing in the morning. I still needed centerpieces for the tables and balloons for the mailbox. My original dream was to have bride and groom sky dancers in the front yard. Remember how much we fell in love with those air blown, dancing, balloon type creatures we first saw at the 1996 Atlanta Olympic Games opening ceremony, Mom? We both said we could stare and smile at the free form movement of those happy dancers forever. I thought that would be so cool on the front yard to mark the event location. Renting the sky dancers was unbelievably expensive, and I couldn't find a local dealer. Silver and white, heart shaped helium balloons would have to do. I also bought a bubble machine to place on top of the mailbox to shoot bubbles in the air to mingle with the balloons. The table centerpieces I picked up contained an earthy display of greenery and flowers in a shallow bowl.

Steve was up preparing ice containers for all the bottles of water, soda, beer, champagne, and wine we purchased. Remember the seventeen foot aluminum canoe that resides under our deck? I thought it would make a perfect bottled drink receptacle. Steve was hesitant, questioning the tackiness of my idea. When we made the proposal to Bonnie and Joe, they thought it was great. Lots of people commented on the excellent use of materials on hand. We displayed more traditional copper tubs, containing the wine and champagne bottles, along with glassware, on white linen covered tables.

The girls created their flower bouquets first thing in the morning, and no professional could have done better. A couple of them relished arranging the yard decor. They wrapped ribbon and tulle around banisters to create a romantic setting. The extra flowers found their way into birdhouses and onto fence posts. They scattered rose petals down the brick path that would lead Bonnie to Joe waiting on the deck below. I could picture you in those moments, Mom, sitting on the floor with the girls creating flower bouquets, scrambling through the yard with flowers in your arms. Your laughter would have easily melded with the laughter of youth. The girls would have been impressed by your artistic eye and talent. Bonnie and I would have exchanged a prideful glance and grin watching you fully engaged in the fun.

Right before the noon hour, the women set off to the salon with a couple of bottles of champagne and orange juice. Hair and nails have become the wedding day standard, a sort of bonding ritual. I was honored to be included and enjoyed witnessing the initial stage of primping for the big day. Mom, your down-to-earth daughter even got her first pedicure.

When we returned in the afternoon with our big hair and colorful nails, the caterers and DJ were setting up. Steve and I couldn't help but be sucked into the middle of all the organization; there were directions to give and questions to answer. The girls went upstairs to giggle and continue primping with makeup brushes and little containers of creams, glitters, and blushing colors. There were bottles and bags and towels and bras and jammies and jeans thrown all over the place. The mess was beautiful. The photographer had appeared and was running around with amusement capturing it all. Steve and I cleaned up and dressed minutes before guests began arriving.

It was show time. Bonnie was beautiful. Lee was handsome. Mom, you would have burst with pride at your grandchildren. The quartet was playing. The guests were strolling on the bricks looking out over the forest. The dogs were locked upstairs in the bonus room. The main players were gathered on the screened-in porch above the patio preparing for their entrance.

We had chairs for the grandparents and the wedding party to sit on during the short ceremony. The rest of the guests had to stand. The parents of the bride and groom were to sit on the benches that formed two sides of that wonderful lower deck perched on the side of the hill overlooking the green woods. Scott, Bonnie, and Joe would stand on that deck, the huge trees forming the backdrop to their promises of love.

Pachelbel's Canon in D minor began as the groomsmen walked Steve's mom, Grandma Kate, and Dad's wife, Grandma Doris, to their seats first. Their dates, Doris's being your ex-husband, followed behind. Then, Joe's mom and step dad walked down the stairs together. I walked down on Lee's arm, a fine moment indeed. The procession of bridesmaids and groomsmen followed. There were nine couples. Bonnie and Joe are rich with good friends. One of my favorite memories of this whole occasion was watching the interactions of all those youthful, witty, and energetic kids. They so enjoyed themselves every step of the way, Mom.

The volume level of the music increased, and all eyes fell on Steve and Bonnie. Father and daughter walked down the stairs, and everyone witnessed the exceptionality of this passage. Bonnie's bridesmaids had lined the walkway to the lower deck before they took their seats. Bonnie stopped to face each bridesmaid. She was handed a white spray rose stem from each of their bouquets of red spray roses. The bridal bouquet was slowly created with each step. When she reached the deck, I met her with a white ribbon and tied the bouquet together. It was a brilliant arrangement.

Steve and I both hugged our daughter and turned her over to Joe. The wedding party and immediate family sat down. It was wonderful to be so close to Joe's parents and the enchanted couple during the entire ceremony. Scott began eloquently. He welcomed all to this happy event. Mark and Debbie played and sang "The Wedding Song" beautifully. Bonnie and Joe had carefully chosen the vows they wanted to recite to each other and expressed them with confidence and joy. They decided on the traditional ring ceremony as well. Scott read a nature inspired verse I found in my book of life prayers from around the world. He pronounced them husband and wife.

Scott invited everyone to enjoy the refreshments as Bonnie and Joe entered the woods to partake in some unbelievably gorgeous shots by the photographer. Most of us up on the brick patio grabbed a glass of wine or a beer to return the nerves to a calmer place. I tried to mingle with all my favorite friends and relatives. The appetizers of coconut shrimp, toasted cheese ravioli, and pecan crab cakes were passed. The quartet continued to play.

When Bonnie and Joe returned a short time later, the parents were prepared to give a toast. This was when I knew I was going to say something about you, Mom. I had planned my speech often in the wee hours of sleepless nights. Steve began with a welcome. He had practiced what he was going to say with me many times too; you know how nervous he gets. Joe's mom spoke next, giving a meaningful tribute to Joe's father who had passed away from cancer about five years earlier. She and I had talked about honoring the people so important to the bride and groom who were gone and would be missed on the day of celebration. That's you, Mom. When it was my turn, I started with the Lucille story.

"Many of you know that Bonnie's middle name is Lucille. But you might not know that she is the fourth Lucille. I am Candace Lucille, my mom was Joan Lucille, and her mom was Margaret Lucille. Joe, you really don't have a choice when it comes time for baby girl middle names. Well, Bonnie had the privilege of knowing both her grandma and great grandma for the majority of her life. She said good-bye to her great grandma when she was sixteen. She said good bye to Grandma Joan just two months ago."

It was at that moment that my voice started to crack. I felt Steve's hand rest on my back, and my strength resumed.

"Grandma Joan would have loved this day so much. She was the life of every party. When you see Bonnie throw both of her arms up in the air, framing an ecstatically happy face, she has just completed a Grandma Joan move. Joan brought joy to every gathering. People truly loved her company. Bonnie, today she would have told you how beautiful you look and how happy she is for you. Joe, she would have called you a gem. Some of you remember that was the expression she coined for Steve when he entered my life."

I looked at Bonnie and Joe while I said those last few words, and I saw Bonnie's face working hard to restrain the tears. I saw her head slowly lean and nestle onto Joe's shoulder for comfort, and I thought to myself how right that looked. I hoped she would find comfort there for many years to come. Life's load is easier to bear when a place of comfort is within reach. I concluded by asking everyone to raise his or her glass and drink to Joanie, one sorely missed human being.

The dinner line came next. We selected a buffet of beef tenderloin, chicken breast stuffed with apples and brie, mashed potato bar, salad on a stick, and of course, Steve's favorite grilled vegetables. I passed the microphone to the DJ and turned around. I looked right at my brother Scott and realized that I completely forgot to thank him for his fantastic job of officiating. I needed to publicly acknowledge the whole significance of it all. All my thoughts while I pictured myself giving a toast that day were on you, Mom. I guess since I had succeeded, my head cleared. I grabbed the microphone back and told the guests that I needed their attention once more.

"I forgot something! How amazing is it that my own brother married Joe and Bonnie! Some of you may not know Scott, but Bonnie's uncle performed the ceremony. And not only that, Bonnie's other uncle, Mark, along with (pause) the mother of his children, performed "The Wedding Song," the same song they played and sang in my marriage ceremony to Steve twenty-five years ago! This is quite the family affair. And one more thing, there are two bathrooms, one at the top of the basement stairs and one at the top of the front door stairs." My head was clearing, and practical details were returning. "Ya'll have a good time!"

I didn't want to say Mark and his ex-wife sang the song, Mom. I only hesitated for a second and amazingly enough came up with Mark and the mother of his children. I was pleased with myself. I could have my second glass of wine.

During dinner the DJ played some special song selections. I thought of this really good idea to try and create a personal experience for some of our close guests. The DJ played the first dance songs from the weddings of family members and friends. A lot of the couples put down their forks and got up and danced right there between the tables when they heard their song.

It was also during dinner that the first minor mishap occurred. Someone whispered to Steve that the toilet was stopped up. Steve and one of his trusted and talented friends quickly took care of the problem.

After dinner, Bonnie and Joe entertained everyone with their first dance outside under the canopy of lights. Snow Patrol's "Chasing Cars" was a song they liked that played on the radio during the time in which they fell in love. Well, this was the moment of the second minor mishap. The caterers were busy plugging in the coffee urns, and the power failed. The music stopped, and the lights went out. Everyone started laughing and clapping, including the bride and groom. Steve and a trusted and talented relative started switching circuit breakers and unplugging cords. The music and lights came back on only to fail one more time for the dancing bride and groom. The culprit was discovered, and we changed the location of the coffee station. The imperfect interruptions to the perfect evening mirror life, don't they Mom? I'm glad we all could laugh through them.

Bonnie and Joe finished the on again, off again dance. We moved the dancing into the basement for the father daughter dance. Steve and Bonnie chose Michael Buble's version of "The Way You Look Tonight." While they swayed together, I knew Steve was working hard to keep his tears in check. We had talked one late night in bed about the moments that would be the most emotional, this dance being one. He managed to look dashing, only succumbing to misty eyes. After a few minutes into their dance, the DJ invited all the fathers and daughters to join in with Steve and Bonnie. I loved that effect too. I danced with Dad and enjoyed watching the happiness of both the young and old father daughter couples.

The mother son dance immediately followed. Joe picked the newer ukulele version of "What a Wonderful Life/Somewhere over the Rainbow." Mom and son radiated joy. Again, after a few minutes into the song, the DJ invited all the mothers and sons to join in. I savored my dance with Lee this time and took pleasure in watching all the varieties of mothers and sons on the dance floor, the young and the old. Steve danced with his mom, which made her evening. You would have had to split your time between Scott and Mark, Mom.

The dancing continued under colorful lights and the disco ball. The DJ knew just how to mix it up. He played a jitterbug song for Dad and Doris to rule the dance floor. While growing up, I remember watching you and Dad jitterbugging on many occasions. He played some slow love songs for everyone, some disco for my age friends, and lots of hip-hop for the young crowd. We interspersed the dancing with all the wedding day traditions. Bonnie and Joe cut the cake and fed each other gently. Joe removed the garter and slung it, and Bonnie tossed her bouquet off the upper deck. Everyone was having a blast. No doubt, weddings bring out the best in us all. But the night had a way of closing in on the party, and it was all happening too fast.

Two of Steve's nephews slipped away and destructively decorated Joe's car. They asked me for toilet paper, shaving cream, and any other supplies I might have to turn the car into a spectacle. They didn't ask for, but found, my flour which ended up in the air vents. Before Bonnie and Joe headed for the messed up car, bubbles were passed out to the guests. We all traveled to the front yard and bombarded the happy couple with bubbles. The guests also received the wedding favor, a little bag of silver and white M&M's. Each little candy had "Bonnie and Joe" printed right on it. They entered the car that wreaked "Just Married" and drove three miles away to the Hilton. Shuttles picked up most of the crowd soon after to take them to the same hotel.

I wanted the party to go on forever. The buildup was so lofty, the preparation so time consuming. The end of the celebrating was bittersweet. When Steve and I crawled into bed in the predawn hours, chatting away, we wanted to absorb more of the magic. We yearned to do it all again and pay more attention to everything that was happening around us. However, we couldn't help but be pleased at the way everything played out. It was a success. Every detail was planned, and the evening turned out elegant yet relaxed, traditional yet unique. The only thing that could have made the night better was if you were there, Mom.

Chapter 2   The Repetition

How do you know if your mother is suffering from Alzheimer's? It sounds like the opening line to a joke, doesn't it? Sometimes, it is. Mostly, it's not. I can't answer definitively. You get a sense. The behavior is just different from the other elderly people you interact with. Everyone loses keys. Everyone struggles to recall names. Not everyone has Alzheimer's. You begin to search for information, talking to friends who are experiencing the disease with their own families, reading the magazine and newspaper articles with the word Alzheimer's in the headline, and stopping the channel surfing when the topic of the television program is Alzheimer's. It becomes evident to you far before it is treated or accepted by the mother. At least, that was my experience.

My mom was the poster lady for avoiding Alzheimer's. Both of her parents lived independently into their nineties. Joan worked a variety of positions at a bank until she was seventy-five years old. She lived alone and took good care of herself and her house. She went to plays and sporting events and parties. She entertained her children and grandchildren. She played cards, did crossword puzzles, and she ruled at word jumble. She could unscramble those letters and figure out that puzzle quicker than anyone around. She read. She had lots of close friends. She laughed and loved. She was independent, very independent. But it got her.

We were close, my mom and I. It wasn't always like that. When I became married and had children, and she became divorced and lived alone, our relationship improved and thrived. Her needs became greater than mine, and that was a much better fit for us. We lived in neighboring towns in the suburbs of Atlanta and enjoyed similar interests. Because she was alone during the time I was raising a family, Mom was included in our plans in one way or another most weekends. We talked on the phone a couple of times a week. She was good at parenting her adult children. She joined in our lives with her unassuming style. She was an exceptional grandma as well, creative and fun, providing undivided attention. Because I was so close, both in proximity and personality, for so many years, the behavioral changes in her later years were obvious and unmistakable to me. They began soon after she entered full time retirement when she was seventy-five.

At first, I noticed the way she was repeating herself in conversations more than was customary. She would tell me the same thing over and over, totally unaware of her routine. Sometimes, the repetitions were memories from her childhood. "Candy, your grandma was a saint. During the depression, when there wasn't enough food to put on the table, she still fed the bums something when they came begging at the door. Nothing was wasted during the depression. One night when I went to bed, your grandma was standing at the kitchen sink canning a large box of near rotted pears someone had given her. When I got up in the morning, she was still standing at the kitchen sink canning pears. Food was too precious to be wasted. And I never heard her complain." Mom liked to repeat this memory if she saw us scrape food from our plates into the sink after a meal.

My mom only saw her mother a couple of times a year. My parents had left their hometown behind once they married, and they moved around the country while raising a family. Whenever Grandma and Grandpa came to the house for a visit, my mom made it a priority to spoil her mother. Joan was so happy when she could brighten her mom's life. She would make homemade asparagus soup for Grandma. Grandpa didn't like asparagus soup, so Grandma never had it in the house. Mom would take Grandma shopping for SAS shoes and a new pantsuit. Grandpa thought women should wear dresses. Mom washed and set Grandma's hair and fixed it really nice. She took her to the theater downtown to see a show. Grandpa didn't like primping or the theater. I guess Grandma's generation of ladies did what they were told by their husbands. As Joan slowly advanced into the waters of feminism, she encouraged her mother to dip her toe in whenever she came for a visit. Grandpa was a good sport during their stay, but I'm sure he handed Grandma a towel as soon as they returned home.

Sometimes, my mom's repetitive talk illustrated her opinions on issues. "I saw a woman in the grocery store slap her daughter. I don't know why anyone would hurt a child. It's a crime. Children should not be hit. What does that teach them, to solve problems with violence?" She'd share that viewpoint any time the topic of spanking came up, but she acted like she hadn't enlightened you on those thoughts before.

Her views came from personal experience. My mom had told me about her father smacking around her brothers when they didn't live up to his expectations. She remembered sitting in the tub, feeling sick, and throwing up in her bath water one night while listening to the hostility. She told me she got it once when she disobeyed her dad and rode her brother's bike around the block. Apparently, little girls were not to ride bikes in those days. Many people have memories of their own "whippings," and some of them will tell you they weren't damaged by the experience. I don't believe it. Many people still believe that the practice is necessary in raising well-behaved children. I'm glad my mom wasn't one of those people; she was quite the opposite. Joan was incessantly sensitive to children's feelings. It's strange, though, the grandpa I knew was gentle and loving. He played tic-tac-toe with me for hours, and he taught me how to walk on stilts. I asked my mom once if she was ever worried about leaving us with her father. She quickly answered no; she knew he had changed. I guess frustrated young men trying to raise a family during the Depression can turn into mellow old men with abundant patience for their grandchildren.

Sometimes, the repetitions were quotes my mom found inspiring. She recorded these sayings or ditties in a notebook. She'd write down meaningful words people in her life said in her presence. Worthy comic strips made it into the notebook too. If she related to a motto she found in a magazine or newspaper, she cut it out and glued it into her notebook. "The best gift a father can give his children is to love their mother." That was one saying she was repeating often whenever family values came up in discussion.

I'm sure she wished she received that gift from her husband. She didn't. She stayed married to the father of her children for thirty-five years anyway. She told me once that she didn't divorce my father earlier because she didn't want me to be mistrusting or mixed up about men. That was selfless. Joan made an effort to spare those she loved from pain. During my childhood, Mom played her housewife role with grace and dignity and kept from me her true feelings toward my father. I learned more truths about their relationship during my adulthood. One day, Bonnie and Lee were little and playing dress up with Grandma's old, fancy gowns in her closet, and Mom and I were sitting on her bed enjoying the fashion show. I asked mom where her wedding dress was. She looked at me and flatly stated, "Buried under egg shells and coffee grounds in a deep hole in the back yard of our house in Vermont." That statement sparked an enlightening conversation after my children went outside to play.

Sometimes, I think she repeated herself just to make sure we knew how much we enriched her life. "Of all the roles I've played, being a mother of small children was my favorite. I loved playing with you all when you were little." She was telling Scott and me this every time she saw us.

I think she loved hanging out with her grownup kids just as much. Because my brother Scott also lived close by, our families spent a lot of time together, Mom as our constant. Joan knew the difference between advising and meddling, affection and suffocation, and engagement and privacy when it came to interacting with her adult children. She dispelled the myth of the annoying mother-in-law as well. Her children's spouses quickly fell in love with her. Mom was just so fun-loving. One time at a family birthday party, right after the cake was served, Mom looked over at me and smiled a big grin. She had perfectly placed a small portion of chocolate cake over her right front tooth, and that toothless grin made me laugh out loud. Soon, we were all participating in the silliness. My brother Mark lived in another state and missed out on a lot. But he and Mom often were at odds. He didn't experience the same sort of healthy relationship that the rest of us did. Something went wrong there. It's strange, when we were all kids, Scott and I always thought Mark was Mom's favorite.

Sometimes, the repetitiveness was about what she observed in her grandchildren. "Lee sure is blossoming into a fine young man. I have seen such a growth spurt in his maturity." She was telling me that exact thought weekly.

It was special that Grandma knew her grandchildren so well. Enriching. But when Lee was a boy, now and then, I felt a touch of apprehension when I left him alone with Grandma. I sensed a tiny element of spite in her actions toward Lee. It was rare, but I couldn't deny its presence even though I wanted to. Lee was a rambunctious little boy, in need of an equipped caregiver, for sure. But there had to be more of an explanation than that to the occasional irritation she directed toward him. Joan possessed a miniscule man-hater trait. It wasn't constant, but sporadic. It wasn't exclusive toward all men, but selective. She adored Scott and Steve. Scott and Steve were non-confrontational men, so that may have been the discriminating factor. This ingredient in her psyche was so foreign, so opposite of her overall character. It reminded me of a new brownie recipe my best friend Lea Anne shared with me. Cayenne pepper was the unexpected ingredient, but the results were delicious. Anyway, I think certain actions triggered a move toward man-hater mode. I guess her experiences with her father, her husband, and her second son carried over to Lee sometimes. It made me sad. Again, it was rarely revealed, but when it was, I felt Lee deserved better. He didn't go to Grandma's as much as Bonnie did.

Sometimes, Mom just repeated favorite family memories. Whenever someone said thank you to her, it would prompt her favorite thank you story. "Remember when little Bonnie stood on her chair after you opened your presents at Lee's baby shower? Bonnie said, 'Ank you, ank you, ank you. Ank you all bodies.' That was so cute." How could I not remember? Mom constantly retold that story.

Perhaps Mom repeated so much to solidify and store these important memories into her own being. Her forgetfulness was becoming problematic too. Perhaps she repeated to ensure that her offspring knew the stories forward and backward. Family history was important to her. The repetition then became purposeful, the attempt to keep up with memories and the attempt to pass down memories, purposeful for both self-preservation and future generation preservation.

The story telling of family history was indeed part of my mom's heritage. Whether at her mother's dining table, her dining table, or my dining table, when the meal was over, no one got up from their seat. The conversation hour began. My mother taught me the beauty of bonding with family through the art of conversation after a good meal. Our favorite family stories proved to be tales of medical oddities or humorous observations. We heard about Uncle Art with the hook arm that cracked nuts for everyone. We listened with grimaced faces to the story of Great Grandma Lily pulling out her own rotting teeth with a pair of scissors. We smiled about our Aunt Frieda who married a black man named Mr. Peoples, and she became Frieda Peoples. We set each other up for family jokes. Mom would ask, "What kind of a noise annoys an oyster?"

We'd all reply, "A noisy noise annoys an oyster!"

At Mom's parents' table, the fun started as soon as we were seated. When Grandma put the bowl of soup in front of Grandpa, he asked her what kind it was. She'd tell him bean. He'd reply in his best English accent, "I don't care what it's been, what is it now?" She'd giggle and tell him it was bean, bean soup made with 239 beans. He'd reply with, "Good, if it had one more bean, it would be too farty." She'd giggle again. He'd look at us grandkids and say, "I want you to eat every bean...... and pea in your bowl." We roared and thought he was so bold and so funny.

The repetitive family jokes at the dinner table were expected. But Mom's new habit of unintentionally repeating herself became more noticeable and uncomfortable. It was a chore for us to exhibit observable patience. On the fourth telling of the story about taking her car to the garage for an unidentifiable noise, I remember tuning my mom out, thinking about other things, but maintaining a pleasant body language and tone of voice to my affirming responses. I'd have to keep reminding myself that she was unaware of this habit. Sometimes, I'd tell her I had heard the story before, explain to her that she told me the story the day before, but she'd usually continue on with her thoughts anyway. Sometimes, my frustration didn't stay hidden. "Mom, I know, I know, you told me this a hundred times."

Trying to find any humor in the situation was sanity saving. My brother Scott and I remembered once when our paternal grandma turned down a plate of cucumber salad at dinnertime. She told us that cucumbers made her repeat. We like to take a bite out of a cucumber slice and say, "Cucumbers make me repeat. Cucumbers make me repeat." That one always makes me snicker.

Although the repeating was the most noticeable behavior change in Mom during that initial time, there were additional signs of her early mental decline. My mom's ability to make a decision was crumbling. She needed a new vacuum cleaner, so I took her shopping. A task that would take me fifteen minutes became an all day affair. We started at the mall to look at vacuums at JC Penny and Sears. She didn't like any of them. They were either too heavy or too large or too complicated. I tried being understanding, and we continued looking after a pleasant lunch break. We entered a huge appliance store. She allowed a sales clerk to show her every model in stock. The clerk even pulled down hard to reach models and demonstrated all the attachment features. We still left the store undecided and without a purchase. I felt bad for the salespeople. After spending the day with a number of vacuums sucking dirt from rectangular pieces of carpeting in well-lit stores, I ended up making the decision for her. "Mom, it's nearly four o'clock. We are going to K Mart and buying the lightest weight vacuum they have. That seems to be the most important feature to you."

We bought the vacuum, drove it home, put it together, plugged it in, and started to clean. My mom put her fingers in her ears and screamed at me, "It's too loud! Let's take it back!" For my own sanity, I said goodbye, walked out of her house feeling quite spent for a Saturday outing, and went home to Steve. She returned the vacuum to the store the next day.

Frustration was becoming a too familiar emotion, so I did my best to deal with it. I'd prepare myself before calling Mom on the phone or going over to her house for a visit. I'd make sure I was well-fed, comfortably dressed, rested, and mentally ready. I didn't need any additional agitators when it was Mom time. That approach worked pretty well. After Mom time, I'd also spend a little while decompressing by talking about the visit with a family member or friend and usually drinking a glass of wine.

There were more early signs. My mom's attention to detail was starting to smudge. She showed signs of a lackluster attitude in personal grooming and housekeeping, two things in which she normally excelled. She didn't notice my new haircut, and she didn't recognize anymore when it was time for her to get a haircut. When I mentioned that should visit the beauty parlor soon, she decided the next day that she could cut her hair herself. She did a pretty good job too.

My mom's energy level was decreasing. When I phoned her during the day, I sometimes caught her asleep. Most people are a little foggy when awakened during a nap, but her recovery time was becoming really long. She would answer hello and then take a good two minutes to figure out where she was, when it was, and who I was. I'd usually get a phone call a half hour later from a recovered mom explaining how strange it was that she didn't know what was going on when I called earlier. One weekend, she spent the night at our house to watch a Saturday night movie with us. She fell asleep on the couch soon after the previews were over. When she woke up in the middle of the movie, she screamed, "Where the hell am I?" It took us a while to get her acclimated.

At this point, my brother Scott and I began communicating with each other more often to discuss our observations about some of Mom's strange behaviors. Scott visited with Mom regularly too. We didn't mention our concerns to her very often. She became very defensive and somewhat angry and hurt if we did. She'd exclaim, "All of my friends and I laugh about senior moments." She was independent and busy, and she didn't seem troubled by her symptoms. She really acted like she was unaware of any cognitive difficulties. Was she somewhat mindful of her complications and just working hard at trying to keep them from us? It was hard to tell. Scott and I just noted the changes in her behavior and did our best to ignore the fact that she kept telling us the same thing again and again.

Mom's all-time favorite, recurring story was a description of a bout with food poisoning. "You know I recently had food poisoning. And to think I bought the sandwich in a health food store! Unbelievable! I'm sure it was the alfalfa sprouts. I'll never go there again. I was so sick for two weeks! Ever since, my appetite hasn't been the same. I just can't eat like I did before I had the food poisoning."

Every Sunday, when she came to our house for dinner and cleaned her plate, she would tell us all about the food poisoning episode and that she hadn't eaten so much since her food poisoning. And every Sunday, we would respond with, "You said that last Sunday Mom, when you finished two plates. And look, you had seconds again today."

I wondered if that food poisoning had anything to do with her subsequent deterioration. That episode of sickness seemed to spark the fire of the downward spiral. I guess it's a natural thought process, always searching for reasons. Sometimes, I thought her demise was due to the fact that she lived alone for her last twenty years.

Chapter 3 The Parents

Joan married Harry when she was twenty-three. Harry began the habit of cheating on Joan before the first baby was born and continued this habit throughout their marriage. Sometimes, he didn't come home from the business trip when the meetings were adjourned. His message was delivered; philandering was more fun than family. His unfaithfulness deeply wounded his wife, and the festering injury bred pus in his children's development. Harry attempted to keep his infidelity hidden, but we sensed its company, not on the surface perhaps, but deep below where the really good stuff and the really bad stuff cohabit. The effect was so much bigger that the cause. As most children do with less than perfect circumstances, I carried on with a subconscious awareness of my parents' issues, intertwining the joys and sorrows of childhood, unaware of the potential power these experiences would produce later in life.

Our household, however, was quite often a place of pure amusement. After all, there are many other rich dynamics at play in the complicated process of growing up. My mom had an exceptional sense of humor which she thankfully bestowed on all three of her children. My dad had a fantastic sense of adventure which also carried over to the children. Mom showed my big brothers and me how to amaze our friends with our "cracking nose." We covered our nose with our hands held together palm to palm, then tilted our nose to the side while clicking our fingernail under our front teeth to make the surprising cracking sound. The results were smashing. Dad taught us to see the world as a playground. Once, while riding in the car on a winter day, Dad looked out at the flooded and frozen farmer's fields. "Now, that's a place to ice skate," he said.

The next weekend, my dad took my best friend and me ice-skating over miles of frozen land. The feeling of freedom was brilliant. We laughed our heads off when he broke the ice and fell in the creek separating the fields. He wanted to get to the next pasture so badly, recklessness at its best. Dad ignored "No Trespassing" signs, modeling risk taking with both the positive and negative consequences attached.

Dad liked to take me hiking in the summer. He wanted to hike the entire portion of the Long Trail and The Appalachian Trail that meandered through Vermont, the state in which we lived during my formative years. He looked at maps and figured out starting and ending points where the trail intersected with a road. Mom would drop us off in the morning, and Dad told her the approximate time we should arrive at the ending point for pickup. We took a lunch with us; that's all. We carried no burdens of backpacks loaded down with necessities, just arms swinging freely along the trail. We drank from the streams when we got thirsty. Deep in the green mountains, we saw trees, rocks, meadows, flowers, fungi, and on occasion, wild animals. We rarely saw people. Dad tried to find sections of the trail about ten to fifteen miles long for our day trips.

Once, he really misjudged. He liked to say we ran out of daylight. We came to a sign that said four more miles to our ending point. It was already past the time we were supposed to meet Mom waiting with the picnic supper. Dad realized we were going to have a hard time getting out before darkness fell. We started to run. I'm sure I was whining. I was eleven. When it was too dark to run, we stumbled along, squinting, arms out stretched. Then, my dad began crawling on his hands and knees, so he could feel the trail. I walked beside him, holding on to his belt loop like he was my Seeing Eye dog. Nightfall in the woods equaled blackness. It was just like people described. You couldn't see your hand in front of your face. Of course, Dad had no supplies with him, no matches, no jackknife, and no flashlight. There was nothing to do but to lie down on the forest floor and try to keep visions of critters, both small and large, out of my mind. After about twenty minutes of discovering the view didn't change if my eyes were open or closed, we heard some friends calling out our names. I saw a beam of light. Of course, Mom had panicked when we didn't emerge from our walk in the woods. She said the fretting really kicked into high gear when she saw our family friends arrive with ropes, axes, and first aid kits. They found us safe and less than a mile away from our target destination. I got a piggyback ride all the way to the car. It took a long time before I went on a hike with my dad again.

Mom preferred the indoor pleasures. She especially liked to share her love of words. She took me to the public library every week to pick out a big, dusty smelling, cellophane covered picture book. She gave me a nickel every time I used a sophisticated word during our conversations. My mom liked to submit funny situations to the newspaper comic strip, "They'll Do It Every Time." She was published three times. She loved to play word games like "pig wig." In this game, the leader gives two definitions for a rhyming pair of words for the participants to figure out. For example, a "kitten rug" is the clue for "cat mat." The leader also provides an additional hint by letting the participants know how many syllables the words have by stating "pig wig, piggy wiggy, or piggily wiggily" after the definitions are given. Mom's favorite "piggily wiggily" was "a vegetable home," and the answer was "celery dwellery." It took us a long time to figure that one out.

Mom valued a stylish house for the family to enjoy. She loved adorning the white Cape Cod house we called home. She spent many afternoons driving over Vermont country roads with her girlfriends looking for barn sales and flea markets to gather carefully chosen pieces. Antiquing was a great pastime. The ladies would come home with funky treasures. Broken pieces of furniture, old barn boards, and interesting objects were stripped, repaired, and rearranged into artistic additions to the decor of their homes. I tagged along once or twice. I heard a lot of laughter being released from those women.

We had moved to Vermont from Connecticut when I was five for my dad's new position with a nonprofit health organization. He was the new state director. He traveled the region, and I remember Mom packing his suitcase for him every few weeks. They had a fight once about the new special suitcase Dad bought. It was a mini bar suitcase. It held a bottle, two glasses, and some drink making paraphernalia. She kept asking him why he needed to make drinks in his hotel room.

When we moved to Vermont, Mom had to leave behind a part time job she loved with an advertising publication company. After we settled in our new home, Mom started working part time at the department store in town creating their print advertisements for the local newspaper. On the days she worked, I loved visiting her after school in that office, looking through those big books of fashion illustrations. When I was ten, she took on more hours and ran the personnel department for the store too. Her skills were exceptional, and promotions were accessible to Joan. But when we moved to another state for another promotion for Dad, Mom always started over with entry level status in any new employment situation.

Mom looked for a new family church in Vermont too. I was baptized in the Methodist Church in Connecticut. She tried their services in Vermont, but she liked the Congregational Church better. Dad and the boys didn't go much. I went to Sunday school and joined the children's choir. I liked wearing those white, angel looking capes when we sang in the balcony about once a month.

So Vermont was ski country, and my dad took me skiing many Sunday afternoons in the winter. It was another fun father-daughter time. We huddled together on the cold chairlift to the top and sang "The Cow Kicked Nelly in the Belly in the Barn" as a diversion to my almost frost-bitten toes and fingers. He let me know that farting while you're skiing down the hill was jet propulsion. But when I was cold on the slopes and wanted to sit out a run with a hot chocolate, Dad could hardly contain his eagerness, not because we could sit together warming up with a hot drink chatting about the last run, but because he could send me to the lodge by myself. Then, he could jump in the singles line at the chair lift to practice his player pick up lines and scope out some new lady prospects.

My mom immersed me into her creative spirit. She sewed lots of my clothes. Once, she designed this dress that had a big flowerpot pocket near the hemline. She stitched green rickrack up the middle of the dress for the stem and leaves and topped it off with a paper mache flower pin she fashioned herself. The dress was very groovy. She made me the coolest patchwork maxi skirt from the material found in a drapery sample book. She was very resourceful. Sometimes, my lunch was a cold plate with a variety of food arranged like a Little Orphan Annie face. She used shredded carrots for hair, olives for eyes, and a red pepper strip smile. In the sixth grade, I won the Vermont dairy poster contest because my mom drew the picture, and I colored it. She called it "Let the Moo Shine In!" It was an illustration of a little girl standing on the back of a cow. She was looking at the moon and raising a glass of milk in the air. Mom was an art school graduate. Many days, when I came home from school, she would be painting or generating some creative piece. Sometimes, she would be sitting on the patio with a neighbor lady drinking apricot brandy and smoking cigarettes and wiping her eyes. She never told me why she was crying, and I don't think I ever asked.

Harry was a prankster dad. He proudly told us kids more than once about the time when he was young and greased the trolley tracks up the hill, so the trolley car couldn't make it to the top on its next trip. He was always laughing when he talked about that day. It was like a challenge. I felt I had to live up to that prank. When I egged cars, soaped windows, or played ring and run, the antics never seemed quite adequate enough. When my brothers poured gasoline on the farmer's pond and lit it on fire, I wondered if they felt closer to Dad's level of troublemaking. Consequently, Harry laughed a lot when the kids got into trouble. Scott was kicked out of college for carrying a keg to his dorm room, breaking the stair railing in the process. Apparently, that was just the last straw in a string of pranks Scott was involved with while away at school. Dad was actually proud and bragged about his son's actions. I learned later in a psychology class that this was called "positive reinforcement for antisocial behavior."

Joan was one of those moms who not only let our friends hang out at our house, but she wanted them to enjoy their stay as well. One of my friends had seven brothers and sisters. Her mom made eight peanut butter and jelly sandwiches on white bread for lunch every day. She gave her children a Dixie cup of milk to wash it down. My mom invited this friend, Sue, and her little sister, Nancy, to eat lunch with us. Lunch that day was toasted bologna and mustard sandwiches, tomato soup, Jell-O, and iced tea. Nancy looked up at Sue and said, "Isn't this delicious?" My friends loved my mom, as did my brothers' friends. Mom agreed to Mark's rock and roll band jamming in our basement. She accepted the noise from the amplifiers and the basement door slamming every time the boys in the band and their groupies came and went. She enjoyed the commotion of a kid-filled house, but she didn't notice when the boys sneaked out late at night, or when the girl across the street and I stole booze from her liquor cabinet when we were only thirteen years old.

My mom was the driver for my friends and me whenever a chaperone was needed. Once, after seeing *The Nutcracker* at the college theater in a town an hour away, she proved what a good sport she was. My friends and I decided to vocalize "Trepak: Russian Dance" by using raspberry lip noises at the highest possible decibel the whole way home. She drove on with patience and even participated. My mom was able to join in with my friends and me in any frolic, and it was a beautiful thing. She chaperoned our ballet class field trip to New York City. We saw the Rockettes, a Broadway show, and even participated in a ballet lesson at Carnegie Hall. On the way to the lesson, she told everyone the joke: "How do you get to Carnegie Hall? Practice, practice, practice."

My dad was stoic. He didn't use Novocain when he got a cavity filled in the dentist chair. "I don't like that funny feeling I have in my mouth from the Novocain," he'd say. He liked to cut the visible mold off cheese or bread and consume the good part left over before it got completely fuzzy. "Nothing wrong with a little mold," he'd say. All bad food was a challenge for Dad. He'd smell it, make a face, and then possibly eat it. We watched him rummage through the cupboards or refrigerator just searching for something about to go bad that he could eat. Rotting fruit was a favorite. Strange.

My mom knew how to run a household on a dime. She mixed the fresh milk half and half with powdered milk. She'd shop the supermarket sales and hand me the green stamps from the bottom of the grocery bag. She set me up at the dining room table with a wet sponge on a saucer. I'd fill seven and a half books to get my new roller skates each spring. These were the metal skates that fit over your sneakers. I'd strap them on, work my way up to the top of our street, and race down the hill, jumping over the manhole cover, astonishing my friends with my bravery.

Joan was pretty. She was petite and cute and wore snappy little dresses that she sewed herself. Her nails were always painted, and her hair was always teased and shellacked at the beauty parlor on Friday afternoons. She used to scratch her scalp with a chopstick so as to not muss her hairdo. She had a special purple satin pillow case to sleep on each night to keep her hairdo intact and easy to restore each morning. She wore high heels and panty hose. She blotted her red lipstick on a Kleenex and gave it to me as a representation of a kiss. Her eyebrows had a perfect arch. When I looked at pictures of her as a young woman, though, a brand new mom holding my oldest brother as a brand new baby, I was confused. She wore cut off jeans, had flat, long hair, and was makeup free. She looked so approachable, and I wanted to know that natural mom.

When I was little, although Mom was very Barbie-like in her appearance, she wouldn't let me play with Barbies. She said that little girls shouldn't be playing with dolls that had boobs. I guess she dolled herself up the way she did to try and keep my dad from wandering because the minute she divorced my dad, she let her hair go white, stopped the curly permanents, and started wearing khakis and flats. I thankfully got to know that natural mom after all.

So I wondered about other contradictions in my parents' behaviors. My mom projected a motherliness that was worthy of a Norman Rockwell painting. But looking back, sometimes, she really was like a two dimensional mom. There was a missing dimension, an emotional one. I knew I was lucky to have such a pretty, kind, and talented mom. I had met my friends' moms. Her example and her lessons were spot on. But something was absent, some connection. I suppose the complexity of existing in an unfaithful marriage, yet at the same time striving to prevent such an occurrence for your daughter, became an emotional barrier between us. The energy required to keep it all hidden must have been exhausting. How do you teach something you are not modeling? How do you accept circumstances for yourself that you want your daughter to find unacceptable? Maybe, she thought I'd notice this inconsistency and think less of her. She never spoke to me of my father's wandering ways. Was it safer for her to keep me somewhat at a distance while providing me the tools to succeed? I guess she just did the best she could.

Although my dad was a fan of rule breaking in so many arenas, he felt strongly about some trivial rules the family referred to as "stupid." He had a rule against breaking open an Oreo cookie and licking the frosting out of the middle. The cookie was to be bitten intact. He had a rule against washing your hands in the kitchen sink. The bathroom sink was for hand washing. He had a rule against wearing an outdoor jacket indoors. Sweaters were to be worn inside for warmth. How do you disregard the big rules in life yet become obstinate over little rules? His second wife told him where he could stick his stupid rules.

Mom kept a diary hidden in her bedside table, a five by seven, three ringed, black leather notebook. It was underneath the sexy nighties my dad had bought her. She wrote about her life with Harry, including his stupid rules and his rule breaking. I used to sneak in their room and read it when no one was around. I have very few actual semantic recollections from those readings, only some images of messy handwriting when she must have written drunk. The cursive handwriting would become sloppy and not fall on the lines of the paper. The writing would take up more space than the lines dictated. Sometimes, I saw the "f" word written. I must have wondered who this woman was that could be so angry. My mom was kind. I didn't recall my mom being drunk in my presence either, specifically angry drunk. If she ever drank too much, it was at a party, and laughter and silliness accompanied the alcohol. Fortunately, kids have built in psychological protective forces. I think that's what was responsible for smearing my memory of the contents of Mom's diary. But the words I read entered my body and hid somewhere, ready to emerge in some revised form at a later time. I should be hypnotized one day to see if I can recollect more.

So it's clear that Dad was a pig, the male chauvinist kind. He chose my name, Candy, undeniably the number one name used when characterizing a hooker in film or song. I always heard the explanation that it was the only name my mom could agree with him on. I guess it was the least sleazy sounding to her ears. He also liked Nanette, Fifi, or Babette. When my parents were first married, Dad had to go to the theater as soon as a new Brigitte Bardot movie was released. Dad only laughed at jokes that contained sex as his sense of humor was one-dimensional. I remember his voice bellowing out the punch line to some joke I didn't understand about a woman and three parts to a wood stove. "Lifter, leg and poker. Har har har."

I sat on the stairs sometimes and watched my parents interact when they hosted the neighborhood party. I listened to the background chatter and the music on the stereo console. A party wouldn't be complete without Herb Albert and the Tijuana Brass. I liked to stare at that one album cover, mesmerized by the beautiful, dark haired woman covered in whipped cream with her finger in her mouth. I think she is responsible for my first sexual stirring. Eventually, the games would begin, games like Twister and Tight Squeeze. Tight Squeeze was this game where you fastened and tightened an orange plastic belt around two people facing each other, male and female, not necessarily married. You tried to raise the belt from your feet to up over your head. The couple that accomplished this with the smallest belt circumference won. Mr. Marin and Mrs. Willis won a lot. My dad tried to win a lot. Mr. and Mrs. West never played with anyone but each other. Another game I witnessed was Pass the Plate. The men formed a line, facing the same way, shoulder to shoulder. A woman, not necessarily the wife, would stand behind a man and reach around to put her hands in his front pockets. This was a time when men wore trousers to parties, kind of vital in this game. A plate was passed down the line, the women passing it from one hand to the other through the pocket and pant fabric, the object being not to drop the plate. My mom passed on pass the plate. For men like my dad and for the women they married, going through the sexual revolution in the late sixties and early seventies as hip, married, forty-somethings was fucked up.

It wasn't what my mom signed up for. She was conventional and somewhat naïve. She was probably considered a square by some when she scoffed at the new party games. *Bob & Carol & Ted & Alice* made her mad. I'm sure there were men out there who would have honored her feelings and actually agreed with her. Dad wasn't one of them. America's change in morality only added fuel to my father's infidelity fire. Justification was available. He could point a finger at his uptight wife and make her feel like she was the one with the problem. I wonder about that now, Mom, how difficult that must have been for you to keep your composure through your hurt.

At the time of my parents' matrimonial union, women's choices were limited. As perceptions of marriage altered in society, my mom, unable to utilize them in her own life, provided me with feminist ideology at every opportunity. My mother taught me to be independent and to make sure I could take care of myself financially. "Candy," she'd say, "Don't marry a doctor, be a doctor. A cap and gown before a wedding gown."

Joan stayed with Harry until the children were all moved out and settled. I was puzzled as to why she made the decision to stay with her selfish husband as long as she did. I felt I would have made the choice to leave the marriage, able to overcome any obstacles that came my way, rather than suffer through such a painful relationship. But then, I realized that was because she raised me to think that way. As a young woman, she was never privy to such principles.

I often question the role of selfishness in life. I think a lot about it. Could selfishness be the cause of all that's wrong in this world? What would it be like if we could eradicate selfishness? Jerry Springer would be turned off when a child was in the room. My friend's father would not have gone into her bed when she was eight years old to breathe down her neck and jack off in her nightgown. A mother would get up in the morning to properly feed, clean, clothe, and kiss her child before the school bus arrived, every day. When I listened to a woman state once that hospitals made her uncomfortable, therefore she would not visit anyone in a hospital; I wanted to brand a scarlet S on her forehead. Can all damaging decisions be traced back to selfishness? Is fear, apathy, and anger really selfishness disguised? What causes selfishness? Is it always learned, or can selfishness be innate?

Yet some forms of selfishness result in impressive feats. Discoveries, inventions, and world records are made because someone became so absorbed in their goal that everything and everyone around them became neglected. Is that selfish? Is it the outcome that determines whether something is selfish or not? Positive outcomes make it all right? We are told today to take care of ourselves before anyone else, to find our special purpose, to follow our dream. So selfishness can be the goal? At what expense? What constitutes healthy selfishness? When does it cross over into hurtful selfishness? Is there some kind of selfishness scale? The opposite, selflessness, sounds good, but martyrdom is so unattractive. Doormat comes to mind. Is the answer always moderation? It's confusing.

My father's selfishness eventually broke up his marriage. I wonder if he has regrets, especially when he spends every holiday with the children and grandchildren of another woman instead of his own. I've never asked him. I don't see him that often. When I justify my indifferent attitude toward my father and smugly say to myself, "You reap what you sow," am I being selfish? I guess so. Does my selfless behavior toward my mom, my spouse, and my kids help tip the balance? I like the way the Beatles said it in the song, "End" from *Abby Road*. I think they said it right. "And in the end/ The love you take/Is equal to the love you make." It's just something I think about sometimes, selfishness, and the role it plays in our lives. I form my opinions based on my experiences. I'm sure other people have different opinions based on different experiences.

Anyway, after we all left the household and started our own families, Joan found herself with more time to think about her future. It didn't include ironing five white shirts every Sunday night. The thirty-five year ride was done. The house was almost paid for, and Harry handed it over. Mom's job with the bank was secure, so her financial independence was set. This decision to divorce her husband was not an easy one for Joan. Scott and I gave her reassurance that we would not desert her, her biggest fear. Even though we all were grown and possessed the cognitive ability to rationalize a divorce, the realization that it would never be the same was sometimes difficult. It was especially difficult for one member of the family, my brother Mark. His own marriage dissolved soon after my parents'. My nieces were only two and four. Resiliency and coping skills were not evenly distributed between Joan and Harry's children.

With Joan living alone, the Bonnie fixes began. Bonnie brought joy to her grandma, and they spent a great deal of time together. Joan seemed to thrive in her new life. She went on trips with girlfriends and won awards at the bank for customer service. She remained functionally fashionable and seemed happy. But in the twenty plus years following her divorce, she never went on a date with another man.

Harry put an ad in the paper for a new wife: *SWM, 60, looking for SWF who enjoys travel, golf, bridge, and dancing*. After the weeding out process of eleven potential candidates, he decided on Doris. She didn't mind that he liked to wear his "Show Me Your Shamrocks, And I'll Show You My Shillelagh" tee shirt every year on Saint Patrick's Day.

Chapter 4   The Forgetfulness

The next noticeable behavior change early in the disease and the next indication that Mom wasn't right was her growing forgetfulness. The customary "Where's my keys? Where's my purse? Did I leave the coffee pot on? Did I leave the iron on?" became part of the everyday routine. Little sticky notes adorned her walls, doors, and mirrors with reminders to lock up, turn off, and switch on various items in the house. She would call me three times on Saturday and ask me to tell her again what time she should arrive for dinner on Sunday, even when she kept a detailed calendar of events on her kitchen table to review at any time during the day. She used her colored markers to circle and emphasize important dates. Her forgetfulness was also interfering with long ago memories. When I talked about a familiar friend or some event in the past, she would sometimes look lost, not remembering the situation. Chunks of her repertoire of people, places, and events were fleeing her brain, and her short-term memory was obviously failing.

One day, when we were beginning to note her growing forgetfulness, Scott and his wife Diana, Steve and I, and the kids were enjoying a cookout at our house. We were waiting for Mom to arrive. She was late, so we phoned her. She said she couldn't find her keys, so she couldn't come. She called back a little later with a story of paranoia, another sign of the onset of Alzheimer's. She believed the man who cut her grass earlier that day stole her keys. She asked if we could stop at the store and buy her new locks and come put them on her doors. She feared the yardman would enter the house to steal something. We talked her through all the logical places she could look for her keys. Mom said that she looked in all those places and claimed the last time she saw the keys they were on the roof of her car when the yard man was cutting her grass. She insisted they were stolen. Well, the whole family, all of us ready to enjoy a cookout, trekked over to Grandma's house to look for her keys. We searched her pockets, the yard waste bags, the lawn, the garage, and the house. The keys were missing. Steve was about to head to the home improvement store for new locks when Scott started looking in her coat closet checking out the coat pockets. "They're here!" he yelled.

"Oh, I guess I did have on a jacket earlier today. It was cold this morning," Mom replied.

I took Mom with me to go see Bonnie at school about two hours away. I was transporting our family cat, Tara. Bonnie had just acquired a new apartment by herself and needed some company. The cat was in a box in the back seat, and Mom was telling me something for the fifth time in the front seat. The cat would meow, and Mom would say, "What's that?" I'd tell her it was the cat, and she'd say, "Oh yes," and go back to her story. A little farther down the road, the cat would meow, and Mom would say, "What's that?" I'd tell her it was the cat, and she'd say, "Oh, yes," and go back to her story. The whole way there, we went back and forth with the meow, the cat question, and the answer. The whole way there, I fought back urges to drive over the yellow line to hit a semi truck coming my way head on.

It was about this time that I said my first goodbye to the mom I knew. I was driving home from her house one night when it hit me, and the tears poured. I had just eaten dinner with her and realized our relationship of two grown women sharing viewpoints, book talks, dreams, advice, and pride in each other's accomplishments was over. Reciprocal communication was becoming impossible. She stopped asking about the new class I was taking or my opinion on a book we were reading. It seemed nothing new could enter her mind, and she was having trouble keeping what she did hold in her mind stable. Her growing forgetfulness was overtaking the strategy of repetition in her constant battle between losing it and keeping it. Any stages of denial I may have experienced thus far were to be no more. I sadly contemplated what sort of relationship would take the place of a competent mom. And at that time, I had no idea how much I'd come to miss the rapport we enjoyed.

My emotions fluctuated regularly. I still felt frustrated over her behaviors, yet I was working very hard to remain positive in her presence. I began to worry more often over some of her forgetfulness that could result in dangerous situations, yet I was trying to honor her strong need for independence. I sometimes felt aggravated when she required so much attention which, of course, resulted in my feelings of guilt. In essence, it boiled down to the fact that she needed more of my attention, so that's what I tried to give her. I was capable. That stoic gene came in handy when it came to life challenges. Luckily, Scott and I shared the gene and the load.

She forgot the route to her doctor's office and got lost. A fellow citizen she found in a mall parking lot helped her find the way to the medical building. She forgot that she didn't approve of fried chicken due to poor nutritional value. We never ate it growing up. She started to buy fried chicken every week at the grocery store and tell me how yummy it was. The day of Lee's high school graduation she called to tell me she wanted to meet at the bank instead of meeting us at my house. She wasn't sure how to get there. She had been driving to that house thirteen miles away from her house almost weekly for eighteen years.

I took her shopping with me quite often. She liked to get "out and about" as she called it, and she had slowed down on her own independent excursions. One day we were at TJ Maxx and Marshall's looking for a new bedspread. My mom asked me what I was looking for at least six times. We walked up and down the aisles, and she would ask, "What is it you are looking for?" I told her that I was looking for a bedspread for my bedroom. We'd keep walking. After a minute or two passed, she forgot and asked again, "What is it you are looking for?" I told her again. My tone of voice was growing in agitation with each subsequent answer to each identical question. On the sixth reply, I snapped at her, and I know I sounded awful. I remember turning red and wanting to explain myself as I rounded the corner and almost bumped into a man standing close enough to hear the words and the tone I was using to talk to my mom. It wasn't fair. My mother taught me the importance of kind words when talking to all people, from loved ones to strangers. She was so good at it. I tried to follow suit, but I failed on this occasion.

She forgot where she placed her checkbook. It was lost. She informed the bank, and they strongly recommended opening a new account. She resisted. After looking through her mail and reading the letter from the bank explaining they could not cover any fraudulent activity on her account because of her reported lost checkbook, I convinced her to indeed close her current account and to open up a joint account with both our names. I took over managing her bills. She was forgetting to pay some. She paid the same Visa bill three times. When a new Visa bill came in with an amount in the due box, she paid it. It didn't matter that it read CR, the abbreviation for credit, following the amount due. It didn't dawn on her that she hadn't even used her Visa card, yet there was still a growing balance. We shopped on that balance for a year, and then I cut up her card.

The bank we entered to make changes to her accounts was the same bank Mom worked at for over twenty years. Some of the people working that day looked at us with expressions of genuine compassion, you know that face where the eyebrows turn up to form an inverted V, the lips tighten and lengthen a little, and the head tilts to one side. Some knew Joan personally, and some had only heard of her reputation. All were saddened to see her decline. She had been an asset to the bank. Bosses loved her dependability, smarts, and customer service. Her drawer was perfectly balanced every night. Mom was one of those employees who probably brought feelings of both awe and jealousy from her coworkers. But a fellow teller learned quickly not to roll her eyes at Joan's fortune because if any teller was having difficulty balancing, Mom was right there, in her modest style, staying late to help find the error. Joan employed a helpful spirit. Her greatest strengths in life were gradually weakening. Heartbreaking.

Our relationship was one of a balancing act during this time. I had to intervene in so many ways, but I needed to be sensitive to Joan's self-sufficient nature. We were in this critical time span where she was too confused to take care of some routine tasks, yet she wasn't confused enough to stop trying to take care of her routine tasks. Before this period, with perseverance, I could clarify some of her newer confusions. After this period, I could manage her affairs without resistance because of her widespread confusion. At this point though, I sometimes provided aid secretively, refrained from pointing out her errors, and pretended I didn't notice them to avoid her embarrassment. What a scary time for Joan. Why couldn't she have communicated her fears with me instead of trying to keep them concealed? It was a stressful time for us all. It helped to share with those close around me. Talking about my experiences with Steve at night, with my fit neighbor on a power walk around the block, with Scott over the phone, with coworkers over lunch, and with Lea Anne over a drink was therapeutic. With each ear that listened, with each retelling of an event, the deep sighs decreased, and relaxed breathing resumed.

Throughout this time, I often made suggestions that she try the new medications that were available for memory enhancement. Maybe it would help. I wanted her to go see a doctor beyond her regular checkup. She met these suggestions with strong opposition. "Don't you ever forget something? Are you perfect?" She became hostile and sarcastic, normally out of character for my mom. She continued to deny that there was any difficulty with her memory that was out of the ordinary. On one occasion, while out and about, we were discussing Aricept. I drove up to a gas station pump in my new car, still working on committing to memory which side my gas tank was on. I hesitated. She screamed at me, "What's the matter with you, Candy? Do you need some medicine?" Again, that behavior was so out of character for my mom, and it hurt.

I asked both Scott and Betty, my mom's good friend, to keep mentioning the new drugs that help with memory loss. They did. With the additional urging, somehow, she eventually agreed to an appointment with a neurologist. I took her. The nurse gave her a mini mental status exam. It's a standardized mental test with a series of questions that gives a memory difficulty score. The nurse asked about things like, where you are, what day it is, what season it is, what an object is, and Mom could answer them all. Joan could spell a word backwards and copy a figure fine. She was asked to write a sentence. She wrote, "My wonderful daughter drove me here to this doctor's appointment today." Mom sounded pretty confident and sane. She couldn't remember the three words, apple, tree, and book, which they had asked her to remember, however. The nurse had repeated those words to her more than once and told her she would be asked to recall them soon. Mom couldn't recall. She couldn't follow the three-step direction test either. When the nurse asked her to take a piece of paper in her left hand, fold it in half long ways, and pass it back to the nurse with her right hand, my mom looked lost. She took the paper and tried to read it. She looked up at the nurse and said, "What do you want me to do with this?" Mom was asked to list as many animals as she could in one minute. She struggled with that. She started thinking alphabetically and then changed her strategy half way through the exercise. She only ended up with ten in her minute's time. It was hard to watch her struggle with these situations, but for the most part, mom seemed unaware of her inadequacies. Not surprisingly, her physical exam was super as she was always very active and healthy. All in all, she appeared in pretty good shape mentally and great shape physically. My mom smiled as we exited the examination room, and she looked at me smugly like she passed everything with flying colors. She already didn't remember that she failed a few of the memory exercises. I wanted to explain to the doctor and the nurse more about the peculiar behaviors my mom was exhibiting. The exam and my brief descriptions didn't tell the whole story. The medical system had a schedule to follow, however, and there was little time for chitchat. Enough evidence was gathered to start her on Aricept, and her memory struggles were noted on her chart. But before she began taking "the medicine that helps your memory," the doctor sent us over to another wing for further testing. Joan needed to get a blood test to rule out a vitamin B deficiency, and she needed to get a CAT scan to rule out blocked oxygen to the brain. Sometimes, memory problems were caused by these two issues. The doctor never said the word Alzheimer's.

When we arrived at the imaging center, we sat in the waiting room chairs until the receptionist called us up to the desk to give us directions to the CAT scan room. The receptionist told us to go through the double doors, proceed down the hall, and enter the third door on the left. I smiled and turned. I asked my mom to lead. Of course, Mom didn't have any inkling on which way to go. I guess I shouldn't have pointed this out to her, but it was another example of why we were at the doctor's office to begin with. She was still complaining to me every step of the way, insisting that nothing was wrong with her, and saying that she had no problems. "I live on my own. I make my own food. I take good care of myself." She was mad at me. But it didn't change the fact that I had to lead her to the CAT scan room because she couldn't remember the directions.

All of her tests came back normal, so Mom was cleared to begin taking Aricept. My brother Scott and I formed an alliance. We communicated frequently. We kept each other up to date with the latest Mom story. We monitored her medicine and helped her stay as independent as possible. He visited her on Wednesdays, and I visited on Sundays. We took turns calling her every day. The venture was more palatable when shared with a family member. Mom loved Scott. He would sit at her kitchen table, hold her hand, and let her ramble on. I would arrive and straighten up her house. He would smile and laugh and converse with her. I would go over her bills and make her wash her clothes. It didn't bother Scott that she wore the same sweat suit every day. It bothered me, and she interpreted my plea to put on something fresh as criticism. I often felt I was the bad guy, and Scott, the good guy. They were just the roles we fell into. They were both necessary. Really, I wasn't jealous of the pedestal she placed Scott on; I was grateful she had someone who accepted her for who she was. I was there to help her maneuver through the messy and mundane details of life.

Since my brother Mark didn't live in Atlanta, his involvement in Mom's life and her deterioration was minimal. Their relationship through the years ranged from intense to indifferent. My history with Mark was similar. I thought it was a good thing, the distance we had, during such a stressful time. Mom used to tell me (over and over in those days) that when I was a little girl if I wanted my heart fixed, I went to Scott. If I wanted my toy fixed, I went to Mark. Scott was ten, and Mark was seven when I was born. In all the old family photos, Scott is the one holding me or clasping my hand.

Chapter 5   The Brothers

Mark was a scientist. He liked to swallow his long spaghetti noodle while still holding on to one end and threading the other down his throat. He waited a while, pulled it up, and examined the amount of digestion present. He informed us that stomach bile tasted disgusting. He showed me that even human gas was flammable. When he felt a fart coming on, he quickly grabbed a lighter, got in the yoga plow position, and ignited the puff of gas. He liked to hold a magnifying glass in the sunshine just right to burn and destroy ants. He dared me to put my finger under the little beam of light. Of course, I did. He explained to me at an early age how it was scientifically impossible for one man and eight reindeer to fly all over the planet in one night and deliver toys to all the boys and girls in the world. But Mark and I could engineer the best forts in the world. We started with card tables, blankets, and encyclopedias for weight. The big card table fort led to the couch or the chair which led to the coffee table. We would construct tunnels all through the living room and den. When Mom walked in, she smiled at our ingenuity.

Scott was a hippie. He had long hair and wore knee high Indian moccasin boots with fringed tops. I helped him decorate his VW bug with vinyl flower power stickers; hot pink, lime green, orange, and purple flower stickers bloomed all over his car. I wanted my friends to see me when he dropped me off somewhere in that car. It was the coolest. More than once, as Scott completed his chore of mowing the lawn, right in the middle of the front or back yard, he creatively left a pattern of uncut grass in the shape of a huge peace sign. Scott encouraged me to think like a hippie. When I'd come home and say I had to do my homework, he would correct me and let me know I didn't HAVE to do anything. I'd argue and tell him I had to eat and breathe, and he'd rebuttal with, "Not really." He showed me that authority was optional. Scott saw me waiting at the corner with my elementary school friends as the sixth grade safety patrol, sporting the cross your heart white belt and badge, was telling us what to do. Scott just told me to follow him, disregarding the wishes of the safety patrol. Scott had on his button that said "Turn On, Tune In, Drop Out" that day.

Mark had a lot of talent. He learned to play the violin at a very young age. He played in a special youth orchestra. He taught himself how to play the guitar, and he electrified his violin. He could also draw and paint beautiful pictures. His oil painting replicas of the masters were unquestionably genius. His creativity was impressive. He stole my doll once for one of his artistic creations. Mom had made matching dresses for that doll and me, and I couldn't find her for a long time. She was hanging from a noose in the attic with her dress shredded and falling off, stabbed slits in her little, plastic body, and red painted blood rivers oozing from the wounds and running down her arms and legs.

Scott's bedroom was the only one on the first floor of our house. I asked him once if he was scared to be alone downstairs at night, not near the rest of the family. He said, "No, Candy. If a man peered at me in my first story window at night, it would not scare me at all. If a man peered at me in your second story window at night, I would be scared because he would have to be awfully tall." Scott liked to discombobulate my mind.

Mark liked to beat me at Monopoly and chess until I cried in defeat. Whenever the coin toss was used to make a decision, he'd use the "Heads I win - Tails you lose" method. He liked to beat me at Rock, Scissors, Paper until I cried in pain. He played the game physically. If I put out scissors and he put out rock, he'd grab the tips of my fingers and bash my knuckles with his fist. He used his superior intellect and greater strength to intimidate me daily.

Funny thing was my mom told me I always went back for more as soon as the tears were smeared dry. I loved being in the company of both my brothers in any form they'd give me. I was so much younger, "Get out of here grub," was often heard. But I never stopped trying to infiltrate their lives. I actually allowed both my brothers to close me up in the old fold up couch that was in the basement. If you lay horizontally in the middle of the unfolded bed just right, with your arms down by your sides, you disappeared in the couch as they folded it up. They sat on me until a muffled "uncle" was audible.

My mom adored my brothers. I remember her sneaking extra cookies under the table after dinner to Scott when my dad said we could only have two for dessert. When a police officer brought Mark home for some sort of neighborhood mischief, she scolded the cop and told him her son would never do such pranks. She told the cop that he had the wrong boy. On Valentine's

Day, she sent them both cards in the mail signed, "Secret Admirer." She didn't complain about their long hair. Mom let them play their rock and roll music in the house really loud. I wonder about that now, Mom, were you worried they'd turn out like their father?

My brothers tried to influence my choice of music. They told me to buy The Doors or The Who. I wanted to buy Donny Osmond and David Cassidy forty-fives. I bought both. Mark played Frisbee in the street with some of the records I chose. I had a little phonograph player in my room that was partly broken. I had to use my finger to make the turntable go around, so the songs would awkwardly ebb and flow from beginning to end. Even now, every time I hear the lyrics, "In the white room with black curtains near the station," I hear it the way it sounded on my little broken record player.

I liked to sit on the stairs to the basement and watch Mark's band play. They played "Wipe Out" and "Wild Thing" over and over. I had a crush on the bongo drummer. I idolized the girl singer from across the street they sometimes invited over to join in the jam session. She had long, straight, blonde hair, short miniskirts, go-go boots, and white lipstick. I thought if I could grow up and look like her and sing in a band, I'd be completely fulfilled.

Scott read a lot. He had his own reading chair in the living room. Sometimes, I sat in it when he was not home. In elementary school, my favorite books were *From the Mixed-up Files of Mrs. Basil E. Frankweiler* and the first *Box Car Children* book, both stories about kids living independently without parents. There is something appealing about running away and living in a museum, bathing in the fountain, or keeping the milk cold in the nearby stream and rummaging through the dump to look for treasures to bring back to your boxcar. I think all kids liked these award winning books, but I wonder if some of us liked them more than others.

Being a little sister to brothers so much older allowed me to be a part of things beyond my understanding. I was awakened and told to close the window behind Mark when he exited the house through my bedroom when the parents were still up downstairs. He could reach the porch roof that way and jump to the backyard. When I poked around in their rooms, I found those tiny folders of tissue like paper with the picture of that guy that looked like Jesus on the cover. I sometimes sat in the hall outside their bedroom doors with my knees bent up holding my doll in place, so I could brush her hair, just listening. I picked up some teenage boy vocabulary that way. Once at the dinner table, my parents were discussing my brother Scott's summer job prospects. He was applying at Roxy's hamburger stand and at Howard Johnson's. They kept talking about this job and that job. I blurted out, "How about a blow job?" I think my brothers laughed raucously, my dad warily, and my mom not at all. No one would tell me what was so funny.

When my brothers were old enough to get real jobs, I was old enough to do their left-behind jobs like cutting the grass. My dad would pay me three dollars to cut the flat part of the yard. He'd pay me five cents for each dandelion I dug up with roots intact. Sometimes, I'd caddy for my mom and dad when they went golfing. I earned one dollar for nine holes. My favorite part was washing the balls at each tee with that two-holed machine that scrubbed the balls with those black, bristly brushes as you pumped your hand up and down.

I liked to spend my work earnings on horseback riding. The girl across the street, Erin, and I went to the stables nearby and rode Misty and Brown Sugar for three dollars an hour. What a fabulous way to spend an hour. We got to go off by ourselves through the wooded trails. Once, we found an old school bus on cement blocks next to a stream in the woods. Some hippies were living in it. They were gone, so we tied up the horses to a tree and explored the bus home. There were clothes hanging from branches, empty wine bottles, and trash all around. It was just like the boxcar children grown up and gone awry. We stole a cigarette from a pack left on a tree stump table and got back on our horses giggling with mischievous glee.

The other thing I spent my hard earned money on was penny candy. The market my friends and I frequented two blocks away from my street was part house, part store. The owner watched TV and smoked cigarettes in his living room, waiting for the bell to ring as someone entered the store. To get to the candy counter, you had to dodge the two spiraling fly tapes. Usually, a fly would have a hard time finding a sticky spot on which to land; his dead and close to death ancestors had all beaten him to it. The whole wall behind the counter contained boxes of sugary treasures, many of which were unwrapped. The old man in his sleeveless undershirt reached into the containers, grabbed the desired candy, and looked back at us with disinterest as he filled our little brown bags. My friends and I loved picking out penny candy in that fabulous store.

Our town was about half Catholic, half Protestant. I was always jealous of my Catholic friends with their pomp and circumstance. They had catechism, confirmations, confessions, and first communions. They got new, white dresses and had their pictures taken displaying that innocent praying position, their palms together under their chins. When I went to church with my Catholic friends, I was impressed with the importance of it all. Take communion; Catholics had real wine, that mysterious host, and a parade to the altar. It was so ceremonial, and it occurred every week. At our church, we had grape juice in little glasses, a cube of white bread, and we only participated once a month. We didn't even get out of our seat because it was delivered to us on trays. Where's the message of importance? I could drink grape juice and eat white bread in my kitchen. We were able to question the bible stories in Sunday school. Mom even told me you didn't have to take the bible literally. The stories were just lessons. Were they like Aesop's fables? My Catholic friends believed in the stories. Traditions in my faith were kind of halfhearted, so it was easy to dismiss the faith as I aged.

My brothers and I walked everywhere in our little town, to church, to the market with the penny candy, to school, the library, downtown for shopping. I walked to dance class at Miss Laverne's three days a week. My mom took Slimnastics there on Tuesdays. I took ballet and tap. The studio shared a downtown building with The Hideaway. I'd always peek in the dark and smoky establishment to see if I could witness some form of seediness. Sometimes, old men would stumble out the door and walk by my girlfriends and me as we sat on the steps of Miss Laverne's tying up our toe shoes. We stifled our curious stares and nervous laughter, fully engaged in the entertainment available in small town America.

My friend Erin and I managed to find trouble any place. She's the one who helped me steal from the liquor cabinet. Once, we were sledding at the nearby church hill, two pink-cheeked preteen girls. A young and in love couple was also enjoying life that winter evening. They asked us to watch their bottle of wine stuck in the snow while they went down the hill on their sled. We quickly said, "Sure." As soon as they took off on their sled, we grabbed that bottle of wine and took off ourselves in the opposite direction. Who would have thought those two cute, young girls would be so rebellious? We drank from the bottle and laughed the night away. I found out later in life that Erin's parents' marriage was experiencing the same shit as my parents' marriage. That shit sometimes fuels actions like pink cheeked, preteen girls stealing wine from young lovers on snowy, winter evenings.

As a kid, I never talked about personal stuff with anyone. Exploring feelings must be taught to children, and the therapy movement hadn't been mainstreamed yet. We didn't have Doctor Phil-type TV shows or school counselors with hand puppets back then. Were we emotionally stunted because of it? I don't know. My friends and I just focused on having fun, and those who had a greater need to escape or a desire to live dangerously somehow found each other. As kids, my brothers and I never analyzed our antics or our parents' situation with each other either. Should we have? Childhood is simply the time when you are adding and mixing the ingredients for your own personal bread of life. The baking comes later, during adolescence and usually a bit beyond. The bread ideally should be ready early in your adulthood, and when it's done, it can come out tasting sweet, sour, salty, or bitter. In some bites, all four flavors can be tasted at the same time. Amazing. One thing is for sure though, when you break and share the bread with people who bring out the best in you, the sweet flavors dominate.

Anyway, once or twice a year, the whole family spent time together when we ventured away from the small town during the annual vacation. We went back and forth between visiting the homes of cousins, aunts, uncles, and grandparents in Buffalo, NY with real vacation destination spots. We traveled to different beaches in the summer. As soon as we arrived, my dad liked to take a swim way far out in the ocean. After a certain point, you could see his arm stroke circulating, and clutched in his hand was his bathing suit. He liked to be in the raw way out there. After his adult swim, he gave us attention. He showed the three kids how to body surf with the big waves. He gave me buckin' bronco rides on his back out in the water. I dove off of his shoulders. I was kind of a tomboy. I liked to do what my brothers were doing. My mother taught me to keep up with the boys, that anything they could do, I could do too.

Before any trip began, winter or summer, Dad had to pack the back of the station wagon with the utmost care. Each piece of luggage had to fit like a puzzle, and he usually redid the job five times. I wanted him to leave me a little cubby in the way back that I could escape to when the car ride was no longer fun. He always tried to. He studied the map extensively to plot out the route. While traveling, my mom and dad and I sang songs like "The Bear went over the Mountain" and "I've been Working on the Railroad" together. My brothers were too old to participate. Mom got us to play word games with license plates. Scott taught me to hold up my hand to the window to give the truckers peace signs. Mark taught me to give the truckers the middle finger. Then, Joan told Harry to slow down. Joan squealed with fright when Harry passed cars on two lane roads. Scott had to sit in the middle to keep Mark and I separated; the Rock, Scissors, Paper game had started with hope and ended with tears. Dad tried to hold on to the wheel and grab the map from Mom, insulting her navigation skills, when we missed a turn. Dad refused to stop for breaks. He wouldn't stop for bad weather, including blizzards. He didn't stop when he hit a big, black dog on some small country road in a quaint New England town. I cried as I crawled over the back seat to get to my little hideaway cubby in the back of the station wagon. My father didn't even look in the rear-view mirror to acknowledge the poor dog or his distraught daughter.

The first vacation we took without Scott was to Prince Edward Island. We went clamming, and the old man with the French accent digging beside me said, "Watch out, he piss in your eye." He pronounced piss like peace. I repeated that phrase all week. Scott stayed home because he had a summer job. Mom told him that she didn't want the house to be upside down when we returned. A funny thing happened; Scott very neatly turned the house upside down. He literally turned lamps, chairs, pictures, books, ashtrays, vases, and anything he could flip successfully over, upside down, the top placed exactly where the bottom belonged. It was hilarious, and my mom actually laughed as she walked through the real life fun house.

While growing up, I remember the fun and the freedom. I wasn't really aware of any negligence. Again, kids are somehow protected in innocence, or maybe it's the naive belief that everyone else lives like you do. It was later when I realized our boundaries were obscure or completely lacking. Inappropriate behaviors were overlooked. The system for dealing with bullying by my brother Mark was avoidance. I was told to stay away from him. When he was inconsiderate, it was dismissed, and he was called the absent-minded professor. My brothers' dangerous behavior was just considered part of growing up. When the confusion set in and became too much, we three kids chose alcohol as the favorite means of escape. Our parents responded with inadequate corrective measures. When I asked Scott later in life why he thought we all started drinking too much as teenagers, he said, "Because we could." I learned later in another psychology class that my parents had the "laissez-faire" parenting style.

I often question the role of parenting in this world. I think a lot about it. How is it that some children seem to overcome irresponsible parenting, yet others don't? How do some children from the same family have such different realities or outcomes? Some people move on, take responsibilities for their future, and heal. Others blame their parents for all their inadequacies, never grow up, and harbor lifelong bitterness. Are all of us able to leave the childhood behind and start anew in adulthood? What about the kids who grow up with an otherwise healthy childhood and make a mess of their adulthood? It's confusing. I like the way Mary Chapin Carpenter said it in her song, "The Hard Way." "We've got two lives, one we're given and the other one we make."

As far as parenting styles go, I wonder which is more crippling to the goal of a vibrant adulthood, having permissive parents or having overprotective parents. When I was six, I went to a parade. I wanted to join in, and I was allowed to. I beamed as I marched along in the middle of the road, looking over at my parents' laughing faces. Steve went to a parade with his family when he was six too. He misbehaved somehow, and his parents took him home. Snapshots of that day would illustrate my joyous face and Steve's dejected face. But the message that rules can be broken was reinforced for me, and rules must be followed was reinforced for Steve. There are benefits and backfires in both lessons. Because I was allowed so much freedom, I believed I could do anything. My risk taking allowed me to jump from the high cliff at the lake but also to hitchhike with my girlfriend when we were in seventh grade. Is it possible for children to filter the danger from risk leaving only positive results? I doubt it. I couldn't. Parenting styles that hover keep a child safe, one of the most important roles of parenting. Yet over-protection introduces fear and inhibits a child's belief in his or her capabilities. When parents constantly manage and rescue their children, they not only steal their child's opportunity to build strength and independence, the problem solving tools of life, but they also deny their child the powerful feeling of satisfaction when overcoming a difficulty unaided. That's the stuff needed to deal with the inevitable tough situations we all face.

Moderation and the middle road seem to be the goal, a balance between leniency and strictness. Parents need to send the messages, "You are capable of anything" and "Think for yourself" to their children, as well as "You are cherished" and "I will keep you safe." Parenting is complicated, or maybe it's as simple as this: if parents don't let their children down, their children won't let their parents down. Good and bad parenting and its effects on the kids is just something I think about a lot, based on my experiences. Other people think differently, based on their experiences, I'm sure.

Anyway, spending a childhood with big brothers in a small town in the state of Vermont was distinctive to say the least. In the fall, we would climb apple trees at the orchard and throw down ripe apples to my dad who was filling the bushel basket. I'd easily eat ten apples per trip, sitting high in the air, clinging to those twisted tree limbs with one hand. In our yard, we'd pile all the red, yellow, and orange maple tree leaves in one heap and jump out of the tree branches into the pile. I can still conjure up the smell of dry maple leaves. In the winter, we'd ski and skate and sled. It got dark early, so evenings were long and spent quietly reading. My brother Mark and I dug a tunnel in the deep snow once from the front door to the street. We poured water down it to make it like an ice chute or perhaps an escape hatch. In the spring, I'd dip my fingers into the maple syrup buckets that hung from the trees that lined our street. I'd taste the sweet, watery liquid of each tree on my way to school. Sometimes, I had to break the thin layer of overnight ice to reach the sweetness. The perpetual sound of rushing water filled our ears in the spring. The sewers were busy with directing melting snow twenty-four hours a day. I can still summon up that sound. In the summer, we ran free. The kids on the street played kickball, statues, or TV tag until moms hollered us home or rang the porch bell. Fearless during hide and seek, we would hide in doghouses, under rowboats, and nestle in evergreen forts. I never wore shoes in the summer, so my feet were tough and black every night at bedtime. On Sunday evenings, we attended band concerts in the park, sitting on our blankets and visiting with the townsfolk. Every sunny summer day, I spent some time alone and thinking as I sailed high through the air, back and forth, in the rope and wood seat swing that my dad hung from the big apple tree in our back yard just for me, and that was a beautiful thing.

Chapter 6   The Confusion

After repetitiveness and forgetfulness each took their turn as lead roles, confusion entered center stage and took over. It seemed each main symptom had about a year long run before being replaced by the new star of the show. In year three of the Alzheimer's story, Mom's confusion was becoming problematic. As her care became more and more demanding, my brother and I upped the time spent at her house. Scott and I tried to convince her to move from her home into something like a retirement village. She hated the idea and insisted on staying right where she was. She told her friend Betty that we were trying to put her in a home. But it was increasingly obvious that her current living arrangement couldn't go on forever. We could visit her more often, take over more of her chores, but there still was the subject of her safety.

Mom called me on the phone one day in a panic. "My stove is broken! The burner is glowing red, and it won't shut off! You need to come out here with Steve and fix this." I knew from past conversations with her how easy it was for her to be confused on the simplest concepts. I tried to calm her down and asked her how long the electric burner had rested while the knob was in the off position. "It's broken, I tell you! It's red hot and not turning off!"

"Mom, sit with me here. Is the burner in the off position?" I asked. "It takes a while for it to cool down."

She screamed back, unable to calm down, her reasoning abilities not working properly. I decided to call her neighbors across the street. Mr. and Mrs. Webb and I had talked quite a bit in the previous months as they had noticed the deteriorating signs in Joan. Mr. Webb went over to Mom's house and sat with her while the burner cooled. It takes a while for fuck's sake. He called me before he left and put Mom on the phone. "Everything's fine with the stove," she said.

The panic phone calls were a part of this next stage, confusion. Her baffled state of mind and her puzzlement on everyday tasks became more and more prevalent. Common events became foreign to her. She phoned one day, frantic about a dead squirrel at the end of the driveway. "There is a dead, smooshed squirrel at the end of the driveway!"

"That happens sometimes, Mom," I replied.

"It's disgusting! It's flat and dead! I'm calling 911!" she said.

"Mom, there is no need to call 911 about a dead squirrel. 911 is for emergencies. I have dead squirrels on my street quite often." I tried to talk some normalcy into her.

"I am calling 911. Oh My God! There is a gigantic bird pecking at the squirrel right now!!! OHHH! I have to hang up and call 911! The bird! It's huge! Oh, God this is awful!" she screamed.

I tried to explain the function of vultures in our natural world. She did call 911 anyway, and they gave her the animal control number. It was things like that. You never knew what part of ordinary life wouldn't make sense to her next. She couldn't figure out the thermostat in her house. She lost the concept of how you can just set a temperature and keep it on auto. She would turn it up and down according to her fancy. Sometimes, it was so cold in her house in the winter that she would answer the door in a woolen hat. Bizarre.

One day, I stopped by and found her climbing up the pull down staircase in the upstairs hallway. She had a police whistle in her mouth, and she was blowing hard to produce a loud, shrill sound. When I asked what she was doing, she told me she had heard the little feet of critters scurrying around above her head. She was going to scare them away with the whistle. She had squirrels in her attic.

Scott had her over to his house to watch a movie one Saturday night. When I was visiting with her on Sunday, I asked her to tell me about Peter Pan, the movie she saw with Scott. She just shook her head. "Don't tell Scotty. I don't want to hurt his feelings, but I had already seen that movie before." I tried to explain that Peter Pan was indeed an old, familiar story, but this was a different version, a movie remake. "No! I've seen that exact movie before!" she yelled. I couldn't convince her. So I told her I wouldn't tell Scotty. I told Scott that night.

Joan developed a new laugh, one we never heard from her before. We called it the Popeye laugh. "Ack, ack, ack, ack, ack, ack," she vocalized when something tickled her fancy. We all just looked at her, then looked at each other, and then joined in the laughter. When her ability to communicate began to dwindle, when long thoughts were too hard to get out, she began another new vocal trick. She would begin a sentence and then lose her thought. So half way through the sentence, she switched to, "daba, daba, daba, daba, gaba, gaba, gaba, bop, bop, bop." She smiled as she carried on with this new trick. Again, we just looked at her, looked at each other, and joined in the fun.

Taking her medicine was a daily battle. I bought her the long narrow box with seven separate compartments for each day of the week. She called it her S-M-T-W-T-F-S box. She'd really say all those letters when referring to the box. "Oh thank you, Candy. I like this S-M-T-W-T-F-S box. It's perfect."

Every day at suppertime, I'd call and direct her over the phone that it was time to take her pill. I'd say, "Mom, today is Monday, so let's look in Monday's section and take out the pill. Do you have the box in front of you?"

If she could find it, she'd reply, "Yes."

"OK, open the M compartment and take out the pill," I'd tell her. She would open the M and tell me there was nothing in the compartment, that it was empty. "Mom, did you take your pill already today?" I'd ask.

"I don't know," she'd say.

"Mom, look in the T compartment."

"It's empty."

"OK Mom, look at the W section. What do you see?"

"There are four pills in that part."

Oh my God. We would go through this every week. On Sunday, I'd fill her boxes with her Aricept. I'd call her every night to help her remember to take the medicine. Half of the time, she had a pill in the correct spot. Half of the time, she ate them all early or threw them away or rearranged them. We never knew which.

Saying goodbye to each deletion of my mom's essence was becoming a norm. Her independent style and gentle personality were being robbed from her. It was a confusing stage for us as well as she really wasn't gone physically. She was actually a picture of good health in appearance. We were on a see-saw ride of ignoring her unintentional behaviors and trying to enjoy the dwindling good moments of life with Joan. The succession of goodbyes was a way to gradually remove myself emotionally from my mom and to begin a different relationship with the new person she was becoming. Coping strategies kicked in. I started referring to her as Joan and sometimes called her Joan instead of Mom. I asked Steve if he noticed this new habit of mine. He figured I was trying to remind Joan of who she was, but really I was trying to remind myself of who she wasn't.

Joan used to be the most organized person on the planet. No one came close when it came to files being in order. Her CPA bragged about her, stating that preparing her taxes was a dream job. Her insurance forms were clearly marked, her bank statements filed in chronological order. She even had prepared a folder that was labeled, "Scott, Mark, Candy, START HERE," containing everything we would need to know if something ever happened to her. She loved to show off her skills to me as I grew up. My mother taught me about organization and the importance of systematically keeping all documents of life in proper and logical order and in a safe place. I had taken over her banking, and I was easily following the set up she had in place. One day, I noticed files started looking thinner. I noticed more paper in the trashcans. Now I added going through her trash to my chores when visiting Joan. She began throwing out important papers, photographs, and mementos. When I asked her about the reason she was throwing away her mother's birth certificate, she just looked at me in that confused expression that was becoming more and more common. The next day, I brought boxes to her house and packed up all the desk drawers and file crates to salvage the rest of her important papers. I found the folder that read, Scott, Mark, Candy, START HERE, but it was empty.

While she was discarding items that should have remained, items that most people would throw away were being hoarded. Mom had a collection of used paper products. On my visits, while trying to straighten up, I'd ask her if I could throw away a paper cup that had been sitting on her counter for a few weeks. She answered, "No!" When I asked her why, she told me, "Somebody made that!" So it stayed on the counter with the stack of napkins from various restaurants, used paper plates, and smoothed out pieces of aluminum foil and wax paper. I found the bags from inside cereal and cracker boxes, emptied out, crumbs removed, ready to be used again, stored inside her dishwasher that she couldn't figure out how to use anymore. She had run out of counter space.

Mom eventually stopped leaving the house. She somehow knew she shouldn't drive anymore, and we were thankful for that clarity she possessed. She had only been going to the grocery store about one mile away and to her church about two miles away for the last year anyway. One night, before she had given up driving for good, she called to tell me about her funny experience on the way home from a church function. It was a little past dusk, and she never drove at night, so turning on lights was something she dropped from her memory. I guess it was dark enough for the police to attempt to pull her over for no lights. Well, she didn't pull over. She just kept going. When she turned into the driveway, the cops stopped in front of the house. They asked her why she didn't pull over when they turned on their blue lights and even their sirens. She just said, "I didn't want to, but thanks for following me home." And that made perfect sense to her. Unbelievably, they didn't do anything, and they just told her they were glad she was home safe. I was surprised I didn't get a phone call from the police that night. Didn't they notice the confused state of the woman they followed home?

It seems people don't really want to interfere in the lives of others. Even when it's your own mother, some of us resist stepping in and interfering. I didn't take her keys away. I wanted to avoid the scene that would ensue. Would I have been able to forgive myself if something happened to her or to someone else? I don't know. Scott and I took steps to reduce her driving by picking her up and taking her on her errands. When she told me she just liked to sit at home and not go out, I encouraged that thinking. She did give up driving on her own, maybe a little later than she should have. It may have been that she simply had trouble remembering the entire process of starting a car. We were lucky nothing bad happened, for sure. Some families handle this dilemma differently and don't mess around with the removal of keys and cars. They just walk in the old house and take away the keys. No questions. I have admiration for those people. We weren't that type of family. We pussy footed a lot. Sometimes, I wish we all were a little more comfortable with directness.

I was surprised Mom's friends didn't call me more often too. She had all these local girlfriends from working at the bank, from bridge club, from the neighborhood, and even a group that liked to go on trips together simply called, "The Good Friends Gang." I'm sure they noticed the changes in Joan. They knew how close Mom was to her son and daughter, so they must have trusted we were taking care of things. I guess, when I did talk to one of her girlfriends, they shared the latest news with each other quickly. I think the friends stopped coming around so much due to the awkward nature of the disease. This was another sad component to Mom's existence that was deteriorating, her dwindling time with friends. Because Joan was single for so many years, girlfriends played a huge role in her life. Actually, they were instrumental when she was married too. Her intimacy needs, unmet by her husband, flourished in the company of women. Joan was a devoted friend to so many ladies, establishing bonds I don't think many people often encounter. I never had the time for such riches.

Anyway, I took Joan on outings as often as possible. She must have felt trapped in her house. She would read signs and billboards and make untrue statements. "I used to work at that bank," she'd tell me when I knew she never set foot in that branch. "I used to shop there at that mall," she'd continue. She didn't go to that mall. Sometimes, I'd try to clear up her confusion, but eventually I just started letting her ramble on about all the places she had been that she really had never been to. I just entered a mindset where it was easier to accept all she said instead of arguing with her about her misconceptions. It didn't matter.

"Yup, that's right, Mom," I'd say.

Joan just sat in her chair and watched TV most days. She called this sitting spot in her house, her pod. Once, she called to explain to me that something was wrong with her TV. She believed the same news was repeating every day. I told her it sure seemed like that didn't it, the way they kept telling us the same thing over and over, especially if you had the TV on for the morning, noon, and evening news. But she told me that's not what she's talking about. "The news show is EXACTLY the same every day. The anchors are in the same clothes saying the exact same thing. There is something wrong with the TV set, and it is just playing one day over and over." She wanted to take the television to Sears to get it fixed. I told her Sears couldn't fix what's wrong this time. Like I said, you never could be prepared for what wackiness spurted out of her head. We were entering the world of dementia.

Mom used to like to read novels or listen to jazz, classical, and show tunes on compact disc. She couldn't follow a plot anymore, and she had no idea how to work her CD player or her DVD player. So books, music, or movies no longer filled up some of her time. Joan used to enjoy shopping and planning for her family on special occasions like holidays and birthdays. She always set up a wrapping station on a card table in her guest bedroom at Christmas and painstakingly evened out the presents each family would receive. At this stage in her disease, these tasks and traditions completely left her memory. I took over the care of her Christmas list. This was also the year my mom forgot my birthday. It was such a little thing, a birthday in your mid forties. But if there was one person in the whole world that you could always count on to make a fuss over your birthday, it was your mom. She didn't remember, and it made me cry.

I didn't really cry very often throughout the time period of my mom's metamorphosis even though sadness was frequenting my spirit more often each day. I imagine one reason I remained strong throughout this trying experience was because of her example. She coped quite well with the strife in her life. She also watched her mother struggle periodically through life without complaint. My mom always told me I came from a strong stock of women. She also instilled in me the belief that I could accomplish anything, and that message was powerful as I dealt with her disease.

I think Joan just sat in her pod or walked around her house searching for things all day. She looked at magazine pictures and slept a lot in the daytime, waiting for Scott or me to come for a visit. Our visits were increasing in frequency and duration. We took turns almost every day. Scott began doing her grocery shopping. I began doing her vacuuming and cleaning her bathrooms. He was doing her yard work. I was doing her errands. He took her to church. I took her to appointments. We both checked food expiration dates because she didn't. Now and then, you would arrive and find food out on the counter for who knows how long. Her negligence was spurring on more family conversations about assisted living.

It sounds so neglectful remembering how bad she was and still living on her own at that time. We all worried about her safety, and we wanted her to move. But Joan was as stubborn as they come. She flat out refused to consider moving from her home. She would go into the same spiel every time we brought up the subject. "This is my home. I love my home. I'm safe here. I have good neighbors. I'm not leaving." Perhaps the knowledge of her limitations in maneuvering through the unfamiliar was just too much for her. But because of the aforementioned occurrences, Scott and I began looking for alternative living arrangements without her blessings.

We asked a few of her friends to help us talk to her about the subject of moving. We all tried to diminish her fears. She had friends all over the country, and some had already moved to retirement locations. We asked a few of them to call Joan and express to her how giving up their old home was a wise choice. Many were worried about her. Joan grew up in the Buffalo, NY area. That's where Joan and Harry met and married. She had friends from that point in her life as well as all the other places she called home. Joan and Harry lived in Colorado and Wisconsin for brief periods early in their marriage, upstate New York, Connecticut, and Vermont for the majority of their marriage, and then Georgia where they ended their marriage. Mom made lasting and lifetime friendships wherever she lived. The moves always began the same, a new job for Harry and upheaval for Joan.

Chapter 7 The South

We moved to Georgia when I was thirteen. The boys stayed in Vermont, Mark in college and Scott working. Harry advanced to Southeast Regional Coordinator in his nonprofit health organization. This move would be the most difficult transition yet for Joan. First, she was leaving her boys behind, and second, she was leaving the northeast, the place she had called home for the majority of her life. The South was far away.

The Welcome Wagon lady came to call when the boxes were still piled about. My mom was thrilled. The woman walked in and commented on the antiques displayed in our home. "My, my, don't ya'll have some of the most beautiful pieces of furniture. They're lovely. We used to have antiques like this in the South till the damn Yankees came down and burned Atlanta to the ground. Now, where did ya'll say you were from?" It was a selective welcome from the Welcome Wagon lady.

I met my first friend that same week. I was cutting the front yard grass. A girl walked by and asked, "Your Daddy lets you cut the grass?"

"My daddy makes me cut the grass," I told her.

"Where ya'll from?" she asked.

The word ya'll drove my mom crazy. When she heard my new friend, Fran, use it twice in one sentence, she about flipped. My new friends and I were hanging out in my bedroom one afternoon discussing what we were going to wear to school the next day. It was going to be a cold morning at the bus stop. Fran asked, "Ya'll going to wear ya'll's coats tomorrow?" I heard my mom groan from the kitchen.

Girls were different in the South. They carried purses. They wore high waisted, tight jeans that were made for girls, not army pants and painter's pants, the fashions I left behind in Vermont. They plucked their eyebrows. One afternoon, I went over to Fran's house. She and another girl in the neighborhood made me lay on the bed. They each took an opposite side of the bed, and they each had a pair of tweezers in their hands. When I came home, my mom screamed, "What happened to your eyebrows? You have a semi colon on your forehead!"

The beauty queen mentality flourished in the high school. Girls combed their hair in class. One girl even put pink foam curlers in her hair during English, so she would be fresh and pretty when her boyfriend picked her up at the door after class. Right before the bell, the compacts came out of the purses, and lip-gloss was applied. I was a fish out of water. I liked to get all ready for school the night before. I even put on my school clothes and lay still under the covers all night. I had my alarm set for five minutes before the bus arrived. I brushed my teeth and ran out the door.

I did brush my hair in class one time. I was sitting in the back of the English classroom leaning against the wall on two legs of my chair. The wall was one of those carpet covered, portable walls popular in the seventies when open classrooms were the progressive idea. Teachers always kept the walls closed, not fond of the open classroom format, frustrated at the poor acoustics as the noise from the adjoining room competed with their lessons. There was a lot of static in the air that winter day. I noticed my hair was flyaway and sticking to the wall as I leaned back. I decided to get out my brush and sweep my hair against the wall in a fan like design, straight up in all directions. I had long hair, and it was now stuck to the wall, radiating around my head like a lion's mane. Wild. Kids started looking, giggling, and tapping each other to look to the back of the room at Candy. The teacher tried to ignore me as long as she could. Nothing made me happier than to make kids laugh and make teachers shake their heads.

My mom didn't find a church to go to in the South right away. In fact, that took years. There was a lot of Gee Zhuz this and Gee Zhuz that going on. Everyone was talking about being born again, going to hell, and all that. One of my new saved friends explained to me how her body was God's temple; therefore, she would wait to have sex until marriage. She was the first of us to lose her virginity. I started noticing those kinds of inconsistencies, and I looked for and found lots of super religious folks not following the commandments. It's probably a bad habit. My friend Fran was a Catholic though. She accepted the fact that she was Catholic and I wasn't as easily as the fact that she had brown eyes and I had blue. I found that Catholic friends never made me feel like I was wrong or misguided because I wasn't Catholic. Baptists did that to me, always trying to convert me. I didn't care for it.

Fran and I babysat together quite often while we were in high school. We weren't very good at it. We played this terrible prank on some little kids. *The Bionic Woman* was a popular TV show that particular year. I was diagnosed with scoliosis that same year. Treatment included a back brace. Luckily for me, a new, plastic, form fitting brace had just replaced the metal, up to your chin, Milwaukee brace, more commonly known for scoliosis. Baggy clothing easily hid this new brace style. Well, we opened up my brace and wrapped aluminum foil around my torso underneath. We told the little kids that I was the bionic woman. They could knock on my hard torso to find the proof. Then, we opened my brace to reveal my metal insides. We never were asked to babysit at that house again.

Another friend from the neighborhood, Sheri, shared the belief with me that a brain seeking recess activities as often as possible in life was a good thing. Sheri was in a lot of my classes. In biology, we came up with this great plan. While dissecting a mouse, we sneakily snipped off the prime parts, the tail, an ear, and a wee paw. We put the cute appendages in a plastic baggy to later place in perfect positions on Fran's lunch tray. We were so proud of our fabulous prank. Unfortunately, as we were leaving class, our biology teacher was standing at the door with her hand outstretched. I guess we needed to work on our poker faces.

I loved that Biology teacher. She was a teacher who respected kids, so she earned my respect. I took Anatomy the following year just to be in her class again. When it was time to dissect cats, she ordered a rabbit for me because she knew I was a cat lover. That was nice. While exploring the digestive system, she informed us of the long length of the cat's small intestine, five feet. As she was busy making rounds to check on the progress of my classmates, I was busy untangling and slicing the membranes of my rabbit's small intestine, so I could stretch it out straight for measurement. After my success at that duty, our teacher turned around just in time to see me showing my classmates that I could jump rope with a rabbit's small intestine. She tried not to laugh with the rest of the class. She didn't send me to the principal or anything.

My new southern high school still practiced corporal punishment. That blew my parents' minds. Progressive, educated New Englanders gave up corporal punishment decades before. I didn't tell Mom and Dad until years later that I received three licks, as they called them, at school one day. The school dress code did not allow shorts to be worn in the late seventies. Many of us planned on wearing shorts on the last day of school. Shorts and water guns were the secretive plan for us rebels. Well, old Mr. Jones, the assistant principal, called me into his office to face my punishment. In my tiny and tight gym shorts, I had to bend over and place my hands on his desk while he took a paddle to my ass. That's some sort of sick.

So our abbreviated family of three eventually adjusted to the south, each in our own way. My new teenage life and trouble-making went unnoticed for the most part. My dad was out of town on business trips a lot. My mom was preoccupied, I guess. We didn't spend a lot of time together. You would think that by suddenly becoming the only child, our bonds would strengthen. I don't believe either of my parents was comfortable with my new female adolescent role. Dad was obviously more in tune with his little girl hiking and skiing partner. When you only view women as sexual objects, and your daughter enters womanhood, a wedge becomes necessary. What a shame for our relationship. And as I grew into womanhood, a time when a young lady needs the wisdom of her mother, the closeness between my mom and me also fell short. It's hard to understand what happened. Did her fear of my sexuality simply stifle her? When I was little, she had told me correct terminology for my body parts and all the details concerning the process of reproduction. I was enlightened back then. But during adolescence, she just told me that all that sex stuff happened after you got married. She never let me know how to handle the situations that would arise before I got married. Therefore, it was a rather unenlightened phase of my life.

My mom and I did have an enjoyable ritual sometimes when my dad was away. On an occasional Friday night, while he was probably in someone else's bed, I'd be in his bed with Mom. We did the forbidden act of drinking coke and eating potato chips in their big bed while watching a made-for-TV movie together. If it was hot out, we even put the window fan blowing into the room instead of blowing out of the room as my father insisted was the more efficient way. We broke two of his stupid rules. Those nights were good. I felt close to my mom. With the removal of the man of the house, maybe she could drop the façade. Her energy was different somehow. She still never discussed her marital shortcomings with me, however. I'm not sure she should have anyway. I didn't ask any questions either.

We shared conversations about our new friends in the South. Mom's attention to girlie detail fit right in, and she made friends easily. She was smart, witty, and attractive, all the components needed to make it in a new town quickly. She was selling Avon and forming new lasting relationships with the Southern ladies. Actually, Atlanta was such a fast growing city that the first question out of most people's mouth was, "Where ya'll from?" or "Where are you guys from?" depending upon roots. Many people you met were transplanted from all over the country. One of her first new companions came from upstate New York too.

Mom was in a department store looking for some new furniture for the dining room. When the sales clerk, Audrey, asked her if she could help, mom started crying. I guess it was just one of those days. She sobbed and spit out how much she missed her sons and how she was new to the area. Audrey listened and empathized as she too wasn't a native and had family back home. Mom bought her china cabinet and filled out the paperwork for a credit card and next day delivery services. Later that night, Audrey called our house. She explained how after Mom left the store, she looked over the forms that were filled out. The address caught her eye. It just so happened that Audrey lived around the corner. Mom found a new friend. They spent many nights laughing and crying at the kitchen table drinking gin and tonics and smoking Virginia Slims. I'm sure many of Joan's friendships included commiserating together about husbands, seeking solace in their similar experiences. My mother taught me to cherish and gain strength from girlfriends. She also showed me that a little booze aided in the bonding process.

Fran and I shared our first car date together in tenth grade. The boys were seniors. The first step for us was to borrow clothes from each other to wear to our big evening. The first step for the boys was to stop at the gas station for a six-pack of beer. After the movie, *Mother,*

Jugs & Speed, it was time to park. My date was the worst kisser ever, so I found relief when he moved to my neck. I didn't think about the consequences, just the instant relief of getting him off my mouth. Fran helped me with makeup and let me borrow all her high-necked shirts for a week. The development of tenacity in the area of love is in infantile stages as a teenage girl. Why couldn't I just tell the boy he sucked as a kisser, and I no longer wanted to endure the agony of it all?

Once, at fifteen, I attended a Lynyrd Skynyrd concert at a University campus an hour away on a school night with some guy I hardly knew. During "Free Bird," a bottle of Rebel Yell bourbon was passed around, going by me too many times. I chugged a bit during the rest of the concert too. On the school bus the next morning, Fran saved me from the embarrassment of puking in my seat. I gave her the look, and she yelled, "Stop the bus! This girl's gonna get sick!" I ran down the aisle, stumbled down the stairs, and threw up in Mike Reese's bushes while everyone on the right side of the bus watched. Without a word, Fran gave me a piece of gum when I sat back down. Unconditional love, practiced through the lives of teenaged best friends, that was a beautiful thing.

Fran recently described the two of us as piss and vinegar back in those high school days. Once again, I found out that her parents' marriage had similar issues to mine. The loose rules of our houses and the secrets of our less than optimal situations provided a platform of reckless disregard for our own safety. Although, somehow by placing ourselves in precarious positions together, we experienced a false sense of security and a lasting bond. Our parents were oblivious. If we did get caught at something unbecoming or dangerous, my mom just cried, and my dad shook his head and walked away, nothing more. I learned later in a different psychology class about Freud's concept of denial, a common and ineffective coping strategy. My parents' reactions were hardly a deterrent, but instead, they actually compounded my habits. I wonder about that now, Mom, how could you have overlooked my welfare at such a critical time? So Fran and I continued to perpetuate the belief that both pleasure and pain go down easier with a beer.

Back then, many of the significant benefits of the girlfriend connection were unrealized. We had fun, talking about boys, singing to the *Grease* soundtrack with Sandy and Danny, laughing, drinking a gin and Mr. Misty, and getting into mischief. But we lacked the ability to explore the deeper psychological meanings of our shared tribulations. That came later with womanhood, and being able to maintain some of the same friends from childhood to womanhood brings a bonus to the analyzing and insight that naturally unfold with maturity. Although we went our separate ways after high school, I've kept both Fran and Sheri in my life to talk to periodically for over thirty years. That's fortunate.

So eventually, with the help of my new friends, I assimilated to the southern ways of girlieness. I joined the high kick drill team which included wearing a sequin body suit. I bought some Jordache jeans and Candies high heels and even started carrying a purse containing that ultra-shiny, roll on lip-gloss that was all the rage. Slimy, wet lips were in style. It was hard sometimes to get good contact with your cigarette with lips so slippery. I started looking and sounding southern, even saying ya'll. But my earth mama, Vermont ways were only hibernating behind the mascara. After high school graduation, I applied to the University of Georgia like a good southern gal. When I left home for school, Joan started working full time at the bank.

At UGA, I went to class and made good grades in all of my subjects except the eight o'clock history class. I drank red-dyed hunch punch out of a large, green, plastic garbage can at a frat party. I watched the sorority girls in their Add-A-Bead necklaces and their pink and green preppy clothes get drunk and fall down. A fraternity boy was always ready to pick them up. I declined the Greek life and followed the GDI, god-damned independents. I decorated my dorm room with empty bourbon bottles, bulldog paraphernalia, and artsy, homemade posters with quotes that I liked, just like everyone else did in the GDI world. Two such quotes, prominent on my bulletin board, were obviously from the influences my parents bestowed upon their coming of age daughter. First, lyrics from a well known Crosby, Stills, Nash and Young song hung above my desk, "If you can't be with the one you love/Love the one you're with." Second, posted right next to the first, was the saying, "A woman needs a man like a fish needs a bicycle" from a NOW button I admired. Dad's promiscuity and his image of the female as a sexual object and Mom's desire that I embrace feminism made for a mixed message of what it means to be a woman. Higher education, alcohol, and self exploration swirled around my brain for only one year at UGA. It wasn't really the environment I needed to figure it all out.

I guess I lacked an educational focus. I was undecided in what major to pursue. When I decided to quit school for a while, Mom and Dad just said, "If that's what you want to do, OK. We just hope you go back one day. We think you should finish." Mom was probably more disappointed, but making my own decisions was an established family condition, met with little or no interference.

That summer, I went to visit my brother Scott for two weeks out in California. He had bought a van and drove out west in the seventies like so many young, peace loving Easterners. We hadn't seen much of each other since I moved to Georgia with Mom and Dad. His little sister had grown up. I matched him one for one on our first night of drinking beer together. I wondered if he was proud of, or disappointed in, my new talent. The visit was a good bonding time for brother and sister, and we had fun.

There were only a couple of occasions or holidays when the entire nuclear family gathered together in Georgia during those years before the divorce. Mom and I were excited when the boys came for a visit. Sometimes, we had so much fun lingering at the dinner table, laughing at Scott, Mark, and Candy tales. But other times, Mark's temper would flare. A blow up would take place, and bits of anger and hurt splattered on everyone within reach. To me, grown up Mark got angry too easily and too often.

So my education continued for the next year by working at a bar. Regulars were an interesting study in human behavior. Jeff was a man who lived alone and sat at the bar every night after work. The bar was his social network, his hobby. He began his evening sitting quietly, a recluse. By ten o'clock, he took off his tie and was enjoying the company of the bartender and the customers on either side. He even went into the parking lot with a lady once or twice, returning to his bar seat with a ruffled hairdo and a grin from ear to ear. Michelle and Doug were a couple who also chose the bartender, the waitresses, and the regulars as their favorite and chosen nightly company. Michelle and Doug were intelligent and witty. They told us funny jokes and tipped us well. They rationalized their heavy drinking every night by believing a little brain cell depletion was fine. They said that it brought them closer to the national average IQ score. It would be hard for many upstanding and goal orientated citizens to refrain from judgment when it came to Jeff, Michelle, Doug, and the millions like them. But I liked them. They were fun. I liked the way Billy Joel explained it in "Piano Man." "Yes, they're sharing a drink they call loneliness/But it's better than drinking alone."

I often question the role of alcohol in this world. I think a lot about it. Where does drinking most often fall on the spectrum of good and evil? Too much is unhealthy, expensive, and self destructive. There is no denying the hideousness of alcohol abuse. It ruins lives, destroys dreams, and kills people. Drunkenness often coincides with ugly drama. It's sometimes the sole reason for a wasted existence.

Yet the portrayal of drinking alcohol in our society is more often one of success and happiness. It is thought of as healthy in moderation and acceptable in social situations. Alcohol is usually a big part of our most happy events. Even irresponsible drinking is celebrated in pop culture. Crazy drinking stories have a way of becoming glorified as fun, and guilt and embarrassment have a way of diminishing over time. People who abstain are often thought of as uptight. I must admit that I'm drawn to people who partake. Is there something wrong with that? Do I seek out others like me to reinforce my rationalizations? Are there true benefits to alcohol consumption? Stress is released as one sips a glass of wine. Alcohol can cultivate deep conversation. Steve and I engage in happy hour a few times a week. When we come home from work, pour a drink, and get comfortable, life is good. We talk. We can sit on the screened in porch under the ceiling fan in warm weather. We can sit on the couch in front of the fire in cold weather. We can sit in lawn chairs in the open garage watching the sky in stormy weather. We stop everything, relax, and bond. I suppose we could have tea or coffee, but my guess is that our conversations wouldn't always lead us to that deeper location without the addition of the cocktail. Occasionally, when kids are gone, and chores are caught up, our happy hours linger. These are the times when Steve actually shares his memories and feelings of his father's death. We talk about our childhoods. These are the times when we express our feelings of being so lucky to live the life we have built together. We share our appreciation with each other over the contributions we've made to the family. We plan next phases to our dreams. Face it, we get sickeningly lovey dovey. It's a passionate experience aided by alcohol.

It's confusing, the mixed messages. I probably over analyze my alcohol use because I started drinking to escape at such a young age. Maturity, family, school, and work certainly decreased my frequency of drunkenness. But honestly, on occasion, I pretend not to see Steve's look of apprehension when I pour one more when I should recognize a good stopping point. How controlled am I with my drinking? Should I feel guilty over enjoying my relationship with alcohol at this point in my life? Is the image of responsible drinking really a myth? Would I be more complete with abstinence? I enjoy my gin and tonic. It's just what I think about sometimes, sobriety and drunkenness. It's based on my experiences, and I'm sure other people think differently and have different opinions based on their experiences.

Anyway, at nineteen, while working at a bar and hanging out at bars, I also engaged in a couple of other unladylike behaviors. I got a tattoo and bought a motorcycle. No one had tattoos in those days except bikers, so it was kind of a package deal. The tattoo was a small, pretty, red rose with a scrolling vine and a green leaf. It was applied to my hip below the bikini line where no one could see it. Everyone asked if it hurt, and it did. The ratty tattoo parlor provided free pain relief though, a bottle of Jack Daniels. When I finally got up the nerve to show it to my mom, she fancied it. Any act of courage on my part was endearing to my mom. As far as motorcycles go, I always liked them. My brother Mark had one when I was a little girl. He didn't give me rides very often, me being a grub and all, but when he did, it was an enjoyable experience. My budding feminism told me if a boy could have a motorcycle so could a girl. I bought a 1975 Kawasaki 400 with a kick-start and a sissy bar. My favorite story goes like this.

One day, feeling very grown up, cool, and kin to bikers everywhere, I was cruising down the road. I saw a group of Harley riders gathered on the shoulder ahead. They looked like they had a problem. I decided to stop and ask them if they needed any help. After all, we bikers were a family. I pulled over, shut off the engine, took off my helmet, and asked, "Anything I can do to help ya'll?"

One bearded and burly guy yelled out, "Yeah, you can give us some head!"

Oh my God, I yanked my helmet back on, kick started the bike, and tore out of there shaking. I was downright frightened and appalled. I reacted like a Georgia Southern Belle. A Vermont earth mama would have laughed and told them to whip it out or fuck off.

Chapter 8   The Move

Most people would spend a great deal of time researching assisted living facilities before they moved their mom into one. Scott and I both did a little surfing on the Internet, looking up local sites. The problem was that I drove by a darling, small assisted living place called Country Gardens every time I went to Steve's office. I loved the spot, and it was three miles from my house. It was pretty and simple. It had Victorian architectural details with gingerbread trim and a big wraparound porch. There were rocking chairs on the porch, usually occupied by smiling white haired residents. It was a one story building painted white with dark green shutters. Flower gardens surrounded the building. I stopped by and spoke with the Director a few times while we were still in the process of trying to talk Mom into moving. I described our situation and kept the Director abreast of the progression of Mom's condition. One beautiful spring day, the Director gave me a tour of the basic facility and showed me the unit that was available. It was small, just one room with a bathroom, but enough for Joan. Residents brought their own furnishings. This unit had a back door that led out to a patio. Overhead was a wooden frame supporting a trellis ceiling of dangling and draping, beautiful, purple wisteria. The stems were as big around as a small tree trunk. The gardens behind the building were more gorgeous than the front. Tranquil. I wanted Mom to live there, and Scott had no objections. We just had to get her to agree.

Mom always fought our attempts at relocation. Scott and I were baffled at times. We talked about how much we would love moving into one of those fancy assisted living places. Scott said that it would be like college days, like living in a dorm. We were dreaming of the amenities. I thought a dining room preparing every meal I'd eat would be heaven. Scott liked the fitness room and pool right on location that some of the facilities included. We both felt if we were Joan, we'd move out of that old split level house and walk into a retirement resort with no hesitation. But we weren't Joan, and we weren't almost eighty and losing our mind. Maybe we'd think differently if we were in those shoes.

Scott decided to take her to Country Gardens for a visit. She was more agreeable when he made suggestions. We had been working at filling her head with reasons to leave her current house for quite some time. We told her how wonderful it would be to give up the responsibilities of taking care of a house and yard. We even injected a little guilt here, saying how we were really the individuals having to take care of her house and yard while also maintaining our own homes. I explained that if she moved to Country Gardens, I would be so much closer to her and could visit her every day. It would be easier for us on so many levels. She would make some new friends and not be alone anymore. The convincing was an ongoing duty. Every time we spoke or visited, we would bring up more reasons to embrace assisted living. After visiting the facility and much persuasion from her son and daughter, she finally surrendered, and we made the arrangements to move her into Country Gardens.

When challenged with a mentally handicapped aging parent, I came to realize that solutions were sorely lacking. Physical ailments seem to be attended to more readily. Living arrangements or nursing homes are pursued for the physically handicapped. The point of deeming an elderly person with dementia as needing nursing care is far beyond the point of the actual need. Most people have to find their own solutions and their own method of payment when caring for demented elders. The children move them into their own homes, pay for home care visits, or find assisted living arrangements. They use money available, savings from the aged parent, or their own funds, until all the money is extinguished or the dementia so progressive, medical intervention is necessary and picked up by insurance or Medicare. Assisted living provides an answer if managing the expense is not an obstacle. They offer some amenities, but extensive medical services are not available. Residents must be ambulatory and able to feed, bathe, and clothe themselves. There is a nurse on site to administer medicine and simple routine medical procedures. All meals are provided, as well as recreational activities. It was a good fit for Joan.

Fortunately, for the twenty plus years following her divorce, Joan worked at the bank. She took advantage of the knowledge she gained and the deals that presented themselves for investing. She had adequate saving accounts and brokerage accounts. Her house was paid for. Her frugality was legendary. This meant we could carry on with the plans for her to move in without the burden of financial worries. We couldn't tell her how much the cost of her stay was; she would have pitched a fit. "What? How much? I'm not spending that kind of money for this room!" Because I was managing her money, it was easy to keep the expense from her. In this situation, confusion worked to our advantage.

We set the move in date for Labor Day weekend. Mark even made the trip from Texas, where he lived, to help out. We usually saw him once a year, and this trip was good timing. Bonnie came home from school to lend a hand. I had spent some days ahead of time talking to Joan about the furniture and decorative items that she would like to bring along to make the new space feel like home. We measured and discussed what would look good in the small apartment. Decorating and arranging was a hobby both my mom and I loved. My mother taught me to use personal touches and artistically arrange color and form within a room to make it attractive and pleasing to the eye. However, her participation at this point was nearly nil.

The room was basically a large rectangle with a small hallway leading into it from the outside hall door. We put her bed, dresser, and nightstand on the end of the room farthest from the entry door and closest to the bathroom door. We stocked the bathroom with all her favorite toiletries. On the side of the room closest to the entry door, we placed her small, wooden kitchen table with two matching chairs, and in the corner, we put a big, comfy armchair across from a small table for her TV. In the hallway at the front door, we added a shelving unit for all her family photographs. Mom and I chose her favorite art from the house that fit in beautifully with the furniture arrangement. Her walls were painted butter yellow. Her accessories were yellows, pinks, aqua greens, and pale blues, all the colors found in the patchwork quilt prominently displayed on her bed. Everything really came together nicely. It was charming. She liked it, and all her visitors commented on how pretty her room was.

The transition was straightforward. Joan seemed to fit right in. I'm sure for any person losing his or her independence that giving up a home is a major step, a most undesirable one. Once you enter assisted living, you're more than likely not going back to independent living. But it was time. Mom's future had to include dependence on others. Again, Joan's confusion actually aided the moving process. She didn't complain at all in her new surroundings. I think she quickly forgot about the house she lived in for so long. She was spared the job of packing up that house or making any decisions about her belongings. I was spared the constant worry that she would burn down her house or fall and hurt herself all alone.

We all stayed with her most of that weekend. We took turns eating with her in her new dining hall and meeting the other residents over chicken and rice. We took her out to the store for anything she was missing. On Labor Day, we had a big cookout at my house with her kids and grandkids. On the way back to her new home, I kept commenting on how close she was to me now and how I would be seeing her much more often. This was going to work so well. She was content. Her obstinacy had dissipated. The worries were tapering down. Now, I just had the daunting task of cleaning up her house and preparing it for the market.

On the nights I spent unable to sleep, my mind devised ways to tackle the house she lived in for thirty years and all the stuff it contained. I had formulated an organized plan of attack. First, Scott and I would remove the few items that were important to us. Then, I would empty one room at a time by sorting the items into four categories: keep in the family, yard sale, Goodwill, and throw away. One room at a time was my plan. I gave myself a deadline. I hoped to be done by New Year's Day. I was feeling quite industrious.

Strangely, I wanted to do this mission alone. I was the only daughter. Additionally, I was the only kid who spent years living in that house. I knew what every closet contained. I knew the stories of all the knickknacks. I knew who made the quilts and the afghans. I knew which grandma handed down which set of dishes. I knew which furniture came from flea markets and which came from ancestors. I knew where the jewelry came from. Mothers shared these facts with their daughters. These items had meaning to the daughters. Again, Scott just let me at it. I was very grateful to him for accepting my need to take the reins in most of her affairs. I had the compulsion to touch all her belongings, to see them properly cared for, and to make the decision of where they would finally go. It's not that I wanted all the stuff and didn't want to share; it's just that I needed the control. I'm sure this was all some sort of therapeutic exercise or coping process I needed to engage in as another step in the separation process of the mother-daughter bond. Sometimes, I struggled with feelings of guilt from my wanting to be the boss of her house. When I'd discuss the topic with close friends, they all told me not to worry because it was traditional for the daughter to be in charge of the household items. They made me feel better.

That part of the circumstances, the dividing of the things, can be awkward for families, but I think we handled it with tact. We had discussed items we personally found special from Mom's home. We had dibs on certain items, and we respected each other's requests. It's not like our mom had expensive and elegant belongings. In fact, she used to tell people her decorating style was late flea market, early hand-me-down. It's just that nostalgia and sentiment are part of possessions found in a home. Scott wanted the pot bellied stove and the antique love seat that came from our great grandmother's house. Mom had promised Diana the good china dishes. I wanted the drop leaf cherry table and the chest of drawers that also came from our great grandma. Four of Joan's grandchildren, including Bonnie and Lee, were at the age of leaving home and just starting out. They all could benefit from receiving some furniture and practical items.

While growing up, Bonnie spent many weekends with Grandma Joan, so this house was a place of comfort and warm memories for her. She trusted me to gather some meaningful objects in a hope chest for her, especially treasures passed down through the Lucille chain. Early on, I asked her if there was anything she really wanted out of the house. She thought for a while and told me the bookcase in the den containing all the coffee table books was her favorite thing in Grandma's house. She remembered sitting in front of that bookcase and spending hours with Grandma on the floor looking through spectacular photography books. Steve and I traveled to Joan's one Saturday early on to pick up the bookshelf and books for Bonnie.

As we drove into the driveway, Scott and Diana were walking out of the house with some items for their home. I gave them a hug, went in the front door, and noticed the bookcase was gone. Dread pierced my body. My mind was repeating the word shit over and over. What was I going to do? The bookcase Bonnie had asked for, how could I ask Scott to remove it from his car? This was the situation I didn't want to experience. These were the feelings we were planning on avoiding. Apprehensively, I told them I was here for the bookcase for Bonnie, the one that was already in their car, that the bookcase and books were Bonnie's request. Unbelievably, Diana didn't hesitate. "Let's get it out then. She has to have it. I didn't need it anyway." Relief rushed in, and the anxiety diminished. I was very grateful to Diana for that moment. Some families are ripped apart over love seats and drop leaf tables, and even bookcases.

After Scott and I each had our beloved items removed from Joan's house, I was ready to follow through with my cleanup plan. But when I arrived at the cold house each Saturday morning or Tuesday evening after work, I was overwhelmed. All my organization went out the window. What happened was haphazardness, unstructured wandering through the house with big green trash bags in my hand. Usually, I'd fill my small car trunk with magazines and newspapers first. Joan had been hoarding all reading material for quite some time. Then, I'd spot something that needed to be trashed. So I started a trash bag. That led me to walk around the house until the bag was full. Next, I'd sit in front of an overflowing closet and pull it all out around me. I'd start a bag of stuff I wanted to keep and start a box for a garage sale. I arranged a bare spot in the basement to pile the garage sale boxes. I'd wander into her bedroom and fill a Goodwill bag with clothes. I'd spot something in the kitchen and start emptying a kitchen cabinet. The format became mindless gathering with a systematic categorizing process, and it worked. When my car was full with trash bags, keep bags, and Goodwill bags, I'd call it a day. On my way home, I stopped at the recycle center to dump the dated reading material from my trunk, and I swung by the Goodwill center to drop off their bags. I pulled into my driveway and put the trash bags in our trashcan. I carried the keep bags into our spare bedroom to deal with later. One thing was for certain, I wouldn't have to purchase scotch tape, wasp killer, or heel softener for a number of years. Joan must have bought those items every time she was out.

After about two months and approximately one hundred hours of emptying and organizing, we had the yard sale with all the items I had placed in the basement. The amount of stuff that was packed in that house was unbelievable, but from what I've heard from many friends with aging parents, not uncommon. We sold some big pieces of furniture and lots of knickknacks, frames, kitchen stuff, lamps, you name it. Scott and Diana came over to help with the sale. We packed up what didn't sell for the last trip to Goodwill. The big pieces that remained, we advertised on Craigslist for free. Some men came and took it away. The job was complete.

The process was hard work and exhausting, but calming and healing too. I must admit that it felt good to dispose of the useless junk that Mom had insisted remain on her countertops, tables, floors, and extra beds over the last year or so. I think I enjoyed the trash bag collecting the most. Maybe in some way, I believed I was disposing the craziness of her disease as I put a bag in the curbside trashcan to be hauled away. The other tidying chores brought order too. It felt good to provide a charitable organization some usable donations. It felt good to dump paper into a recycle bin. It felt really good to gather history through the photograph collections and the meaningful objects that held family stories within their glass, wood, or metal forms. I would have to write down the stories for the recipients of these heirlooms.

The empty house didn't depress me. Although some happy memories occurred within its walls, deep down, that house always reminded me of a wayward young woman existing alongside her disconnected parents. Once I left that home and returned as a visitor, my sleep was always fitful if I had to stay the night. If I spent only the day, the moment I returned to my own home and opened my front door, I was welcomed by a sense of peace and warmth. This finality was good. The relief of properly placing the contents of the home, especially the human contents, far outweighed any sadness of dismantling the past.

During that laborious time, every once in a while, Mom inquired about her house and it's possessions. I told her that her children and grandchildren were all dividing up her things. I showed her the table and chest of drawers and some other decorative items now placed in my house when she was over for a visit. I told her we were selling the house. She seemed to be satisfied with our strategy. She wanted to see her house one more time before it changed hands, so I drove her over to the empty home. I thought she might be upset by this experience, but she just walked around and said, "It's smaller than I remember." The goodbye we shared at this stage, the goodbye to her old house and to her independence, was not so bad. I was so relieved to have the clutter gone and the mom safe. She was too disorientated to be sad.

I accomplished my goal and called my realtor right after the first of January. The house needed a little polishing before we put it on the market. We hired a yard crew to clean up the neglected backyard, a cleaning crew to spruce up the inside of the house, and a painter to freshen a stained ceiling and the front foyer. Our fabulous realtor did her magic, and in a month's time we were in the negotiating stage with a potential buyer. After an inspection, a few more repairs were necessary. The closing date arrived, and Steve accompanied me as I sat at the big table with the realtors and lawyer to act in Mom's place. Scott and I had obtained dual power of attorney right after we moved Mom to Country Gardens. Joan was completely unable to participate in any part of the legal process of selling a house.

Free time was unheard of during those months. I'd stop and see Mom every afternoon after my day at work. I went to her old house every Saturday and one evening during the week to toil away, and I took care of my own house chores every Sunday. Understanding the depth of the labor involved was out of her reach. She was oblivious to all the time we spent and hard work we tackled completing this move to Country Gardens and settling her house affairs. Steve helped me all along the way, picking up my slack, and never complaining about how much time I was at Joan's house alone. He was absolutely supportive and fabulous, and I was grateful.

Steve isn't the kind of husband who brings home flowers or buys jewelry. He doesn't like to dance or partake in public displays of affection. He is the kind of husband who supports my goals and efforts in every aspect of life. He is proud to introduce me to his friends and coworkers. He fills my car up with gas whenever he borrows it. He replaces my soap in the shower when it becomes tiny. He replaces empty toilet paper rolls too. He fixes everything around the house that needs fixing, a chance to try out some special new tool. Once, he took a piece of wood and cut it into a heart shape. He engraved our names on it, cut it up into jigsaw pieces, and painted it red for a Valentine's Day present for me. He used a few new tools for that one. For Christmas one year, he did buy me an appliance, a bread maker. But it came with the promise that I would never have to learn how to use it and that he would make homemade bread on weekends in the cold winter months. He kept his promise. He also chops the wood and keeps the fire going in those cold winter months. He opens doors for me, and he's never forgotten once to put the toilet seat down.

Steve is the kind of man who has absolutely no doubts whatsoever on his meaning in life, his utopia, his total fulfillment. A wife, two kids, a dog, and a house in the suburbs, that is his dream. He's truly content. He doesn't really understand restlessness or people who are always searching for more. That doesn't make sense to him, and I love him for that.

Joan loved Steve. She referred to him as a gem. She liked that he was also Canadian like her mother. She was so happy for me because I found a partner in life who was a real gentleman. She felt right away he was honorable, a crucial personality trait to both of us when it came to me finding a man. Even though she preached feminism, and I absorbed feminism, on some level, we both saw him as my knight in shining armor. And at the point he entered my life, I was somewhat of a damsel in distress. He came out of nowhere when we least expected it.

Chapter 9 The Husband

I drove to Myrtle Beach in August a few days after my twentieth birthday with my roommate Melanie, my best friend Lea Anne, and Lea Anne's big sister, Karen. We were all ready for a mini girl's vacation, and we all left our boyfriends back at home. The plan was sun bathing, swimming, playing Frisbee, and of course, going out to drink and dance every night.

Fifteen minutes after pulling into the hotel parking lot, our towels were smoothed out in the sand, and Melanie was searching for a good station to listen to on the radio. "Super Freak" by Rick James came on the air, and our eyes were taking in the scenery. We noticed three guys lounging next to us, and we asked Karen to take our picture with them, simply to give us something to take back home to make our boyfriends jealous. One of the guys was cute and quiet; he caught my eye. The next day out on the beach, Stan, a guy from our picture, not the cute and quiet one, wandered over to start up a conversation. He was kind of cocky, very tan, and buff. We found out they drove to Myrtle Beach in his van all the way from Canada for a guy's vacation. He found out what bar we were headed to that night. We named him Tan Stan the Man with a Van from Can.

When we arrived at Cowboy's, the three Canadians were already at a table. As we walked over to join them, I called for the quiet, blonde guy. It's just something girls do when they have the feeling. I bet guys do it too. I didn't get the feeling very often, but when I did, I paid attention. I spent the evening talking to Steve, the quiet Canadian, and making him dance with me. I was having so much fun. I also drank a lot of beer. Steve didn't try to match me. I wanted to ride the mechanical bull at the back of the bar. A minute into the ride, my mouth was open wide with hysterical laughter as I was thrown through the air, landing like a rag doll on the thick pads. I crawled back on the machine, faced the wrong way, grabbed hold of the bull's tail, and yelled, "Let's go again! I'm ready!" Steve thought it was time to leave.

I rode back to the hotel with Steve and Stan in the van. It was one of those gaudy seventies vans, covered with baby blue, crushed velvet upholstery, round tinted windows, and a big bed in the back. It fit Stan perfectly, not Steve at all. Karen drove Melanie, Lea Anne, and Richard, the third Canadian, back in her car. We were all going to party some more down on the beach. Steve and I went for a walk instead, barefoot in the surf. I was really tired, or more likely, ready to pass out. We decided to head back to the van to be alone, and I was out in a minute in Steve's arms on the bed in the back.

I woke up very early the next morning, feeling very thirsty, surprised at my surroundings. Steve said he had some apple juice in his room. While he was fetching the cure to my cottonmouth, I was trying to remember how I arrived in this position. The sound of violins was competing with the twang of country music through the beat of a pounding headache. I was foggy about the latter events of the previous evening, but I remembered the ecstatic infatuation I was still feeling for this guy who didn't take advantage of me in my vulnerable state. That fact, I knew for sure. After some much needed liquid refreshment and detailed explanations of our night at Cowboy's from Steve, we headed back to our rooms to shower. The plan was to meet on the beach thirty minutes later. I woke up Lea Anne, Melanie, and Karen, banging on the door. I informed them that I was going to marry the Canadian named Steve.

The night we met, the beginning of our life together, doesn't sound at all like a romantic and innocent encounter in line with the old fashioned, love struck movies. That night sounds dangerous and rather trashy. But I can honestly say that all of my memories and emotions surrounding that encounter are overwhelmingly of the romantic and innocent kind, just like the old fashioned, love struck movies. Sometimes, things aren't how they seem.

I guess the acceptable romance began that morning. I was feeling a little hung-over and embarrassed, and Steve put me at ease. We talked again, not in a loud, smoky, crowded bar, but instead, on a warm, sandy, wave-crashing beach. We wanted to learn everything about each other. We both loved Monty Python. We both loved our roast beef medium rare. We both had all the Elton John albums from 1971 to 1975 in our personal collection. We loved the idea of camping and hiking, anything having to do with nature and the great outdoors. We both had the same crooked tooth. Lea Anne, who was in dental hygiene school, told me the tooth was number seven. The comfort level we felt with each other was extraordinary. We talked about relationships, family, religion, and politics. Our dreams, ideas, beliefs, and goals were the same, a perfect match. He applied suntan lotion to the back of my body, and I could tell I missed something the night before. His hands felt really good on my skin. My eyes closed, and my lips curled into a blissful grin.

We both were dog lovers. Steve told me all about his beloved family pet, Sandy, who had recently been put down. I had this theory about men and dogs. Dog lovers make good husbands. A dog owner must possess a high level of responsibility to love and care for a dog. Dog lovers understand that sometimes an inconvenient sacrifice is well worth the benefits of absolute devotion. That's good family stuff. My dad never wanted a dog. I had another theory about men. I'd ask a guy if he would rather be stuck on Gilligan's Island with Ginger or Mary Ann. If they chose Ginger, I put them in the sexist pig club. If they chose Mary Ann, I put them in the possible prospect club. When I asked Steve which character he'd rather be stranded with, he answered without a moment's hesitation, Mary Ann. My dad, of course, chose Ginger.

Steve got up and left for a little while in the afternoon. He said he'd be right back. I missed him. He surprised me, returning with a silver seagull necklace and a teddy bear sporting a Myrtle Beach tee shirt. Steve and I spent the rest of the afternoon and evening falling in love, and it was a beautiful thing.

Sadly, my vacation was to end the next day. We spent almost every minute together, from the moment I walked his way at Cowboy's, until the moment I drove away in my Vega. It really was only forty-eight hours. How can you build a future on that? Steve and I hugged tight and long and promised to send each other love letters. I left in the late afternoon of the third day of our life together. He had one more night in Myrtle Beach which he spent alone. Richard and Stan went out to party some more.

I received the first love letter within a few days of returning home. It was good. Steve was already trying to find ways to get together again. I read it to my mom who termed our encounter a summer romance. She didn't try to sway my feelings in any way. Mom always smiled at my pleasurable experiences right along with me and never inserted any condescendence or doubt toward the validity of my feelings. That's a gift. Well, I got another mushy letter the very next day. Steve and Richard were planning on driving down to Georgia in September. I couldn't believe it. He lived one thousand miles away, yet he was coming for a long weekend!

The date was the same weekend I promised my dwindling boyfriend I'd drive him back to school four hours away in South Georgia. I worked it out so that I'd be back in town about the same time Steve arrived. I made my boyfriend get up at four o'clock in the morning to start the road trip. When I helped him carry his bags into the dorm room, I said, "This is nice, but I'm sorry I have to leave." I think he sensed the upcoming Dear John letter he was about to receive.

I don't know who drove faster to Atlanta, the car traveling north or the car traveling south, but Steve beat me. I couldn't believe I wasn't the one to open the apartment door for him after his sixteen-hour drive to see me. My second roommate, Suzy, was. Suzy liked to enter wet tee shirt contests. She had mirrors on the ceiling of her waterbed furniture ensemble. She liked cowboys, and she had the mouth of a truck driver. She took Steve and Richard to Chili's, the restaurant where she, Melanie, and

I were all waitresses. We all worked together and shared an apartment. Only Melanie and I shared a real friendship. I found Suzy's note and drove to Chili's, a little worried. I didn't want Steve to think I was as rough as some of my pals.

Our re-acquaintance was a little awkward at first, maybe too many people around, maybe fear or doubt. Did we really believe in our initial feelings? I took Steve and Richard over to my parents' house for dinner to meet Mom and Dad. My dad stuck his head out from behind the paper long enough to say hello. He usually sat in his chair each evening in his undergarments consisting of black socks, pastel boxers, and a white, crew neck tee shirt. Sometimes, the tee shirt would be a V-neck left over from the leisure suit craze. I remember Mom trying to convince Dad that his usual crew neck didn't look right with the open collar style of the leisure suit shirt. They bought him two leisure suits at Sears, one baby blue and one brown checkered, and a package of V neck undershirts to go with. On this night, he kept his work clothes on, and he refrained from farting, a nightly companion to the newspaper reading in the underwear. After each fart, he always asked, "Who did that?" Mom wore her apron and put out a nice dinner for our Canadian guests who removed their shoes when they entered the house. My mom liked Steve. The evening and the actual weekend went by quickly. Again, we agonized over our tearful farewells and dreamed about another visit. Most of our doubts and fears had diminished.

Steve flew down to Atlanta for a week in October. My parents were going on a trip to Buffalo, NY the same week, so we took advantage of their empty house and moved in. He arrived the day they were to leave. Mom watched me put my overnight bag in my old room. Steve put his suitcase in the guest room. I wonder if we fooled her for a minute. I doubted it. We all went to Steak and Ale for an early dinner before my parents' flight. I guess they didn't worry about leaving me alone with the polite Canadian.

That week was unbelievably wonderful. We solidified our promise to each other that somehow we would be together forever. I took the week off from work, and we spent nearly every minute together. I did leave twice to attend my classes at Georgia State University. I had enrolled part time fall quarter, trying to get back to the education thing. Steve studied while I was away because he had to take his automotive mechanic exams when he returned to Canada. He had been in school and apprenticing for four years and was close to becoming a certified mechanic. It's quite an extensive process in his country. I told him that to become a mechanic here in Georgia, you just had to have dirty fingernails.

The ride to the airport at the end of the week was somber. Steve was working on another letter to me while I drove. I read it after we parked the Vega. He had described the week we just shared as a week in heaven. I went home and played two of my favorite classic albums real loud. Carole King's, "You're so Far Away" and Carly Simon's, "Right Thing to Do" helped me get my tears out.

Our next reunion was in Canada. I flew up to the Great White North in November. I enjoyed the snow and cold because it reminded me of growing up in Vermont. I met his family and friends, and he showed me the sights. Steve lived at home with his mom. His dad had passed away when Steve was twenty-one, four years earlier, and I think he felt a sense of responsibility for the man jobs at the house. I found that kids didn't leave home as quickly in Canada as they did in the States. The family unit seemed more valued. Rent, as well as the cost of living, was more expensive there too. Most of Steve's friends lived in the basement of their childhood homes until they were married or enjoying a solid career. We had visits with his three sisters. Everyone wanted to meet the girl from Georgia that Steve had fallen head over heels for.

Steve drove down to Atlanta in December and spent New Year's Eve with me. The next day, we drove out to the country and adopted a little, black lab mix puppy. We named him Canuck. He kept me company when Steve had to return home. This once a month visiting thing was difficult. We were lucky to have such flexible jobs allowing us time off, although unpaid time off.

I returned to Canada in February for Valentine's Day, and it happened, a ring. Steve was so nervous. After uncharacteristically downing two glasses of champagne, he presented me with a dozen red roses and a box of chocolates. He hid the ring inside the box of chocolates. The cellophane wrapper was painstakingly undone and redone, so the box did not look tampered with at all. Instead of a center chocolate, the ring was placed there. It was exquisite, and of course, I said yes. I flew home engaged and dreaming of an August evening wedding. My mom's reaction was predictable, a smile and a nod. She loved seeing me happy. She didn't at all question my decision to accept his proposal. She must have momentarily forgotten about all her lectures to me on independence. Strangely enough, I think she was happy to be relieved of the job as my primary caregiver. She worried about me. She probably hoped Steve could do a better job.

In March, Steve drove down to Georgia to pick me up! We traveled to Vermont to begin wedding plans. As to the question of where to hold the wedding, we decided neither of our hometowns was the right place. Georgia was too far for his family and friends. I didn't want to get married in Canada either. We chose Vermont as the location. It was close enough to Canada, and most of my family's relatives resided in Buffalo or the New England area, also close. I just had to convince some of my Georgia Peach girlfriends to make the trip north.

For the ceremony, we visited and booked the church I grew up attending, Grace Congregational United Church of Christ. It was very impressive, a beautiful structure with a typical, tall, white New England steeple. A church wedding was not necessary for either of us, but we decided to go with tradition. After meeting with the minister, we were relieved that he was easygoing and very liberal. The service would be short and sweet. Of course, we chose the modern vows to recite, excluding the word OBEY.

Steve and I had similar experiences with family and religion while growing up. We both were given the freedom during adolescence to decide for ourselves if we wanted to keep going to church. We both had declined on the continuation of organized religion as a part of our lives.

I often question the role of religion in this world. I think a lot about it. So much of the hyper-religious ideals bring me great frustration. How can people dismiss science in favor of religion? I'm excited about the stem cell work to possibly cure paralysis. I shake my head when people want to talk about dinosaurs and man existing together. How can some turn their heads when priests, who must remain unnaturally celibate, sexually molest altar boys? What about the sexism that flourishes in many religious sects? Women are second-class citizens and horrendously abused under some religious practices. How about the unbelievable amount of violence, cruelty, and destruction during religious wars? My God is better than your God. Hypocrisy is too easy to find, just begin with Jim and Tammy Faye. How arrogant is it to think that only one type of belief holds a golden ticket to heaven? And why do some insist on trying to convert people who are content with their own belief system? Can't we have moderation with religion? When a parent of a child who survives cancer says, "Our prayers were answered. God listened to us and cured him." I wonder how that makes the parent of the child who died from cancer feel. God didn't listen to them? It just makes no sense. After Steve's father died, someone told him that his dad must have an important job to do in heaven. Steve wondered what job was more important than being a father. "God has a plan." Really, why does it include genocide? "There is a reason for everything." What could be the reason for rape? When someone wonders how you can look at a colorful sunset over a grand mountaintop and deny the presence of God, I wonder how they can look at the cigarette burn scars and the ribs of an abused and starving child and believe in the presence of God. It's the same thought process. The word faith actually drives me crazy. People ignore common sense and go with faith. "All I can do is pray and put it in God's hands." No, actually there are many things you can do to change a situation. It requires action on your part. So much of what defines religion puzzles me. It's just so conveniently inconsistent. And I sometimes don't find a positive correlation between those people who prominently display the crucifix in their jewelry with genuine kindness and acceptance toward all human kind.

Yet I must admit many great deeds are accomplished by well meaning religious folks. Food is delivered to the hungry. Shelter is built for the homeless. Medicine and technology are introduced to many areas of the world in need of these services. The church and its benevolence provide glorious aid to those lost and forlorn and in need of safety. Jesus has turned around lives; I hear about it all the time. He provides hope to the hopeless. When your parents abandon you and you have no one to love you, it's very comforting to know God loves you. Religion strengthens folks and provides guidelines. It's hard to top, "Do unto others as you would have others do unto you."

But there's good stuff in all religions. I love the idea of Buddha and his belief of not hurting any living thing. I love the idea of reincarnation to explain that little savant kid who can play the piano like Liberace or that other savant kid who knows everything about fighter pilots and jets at the age of three even though his parents have never exposed him to any of that knowledge. I love the idea of Karma; what goes around comes around. I love the idea of Unitarians, one spirit and one universe. I love the Native American approach, Father Sky and Mother Earth. We must respect the natural world and live in peace and harmony with our surroundings, never taking more than we need. I love how Shug explained God to Celie in *The Color Purple*. There are so many choices with spirituality, a term so popular today. Sometimes, I wonder what it would feel like to be so sure with one belief, to embrace one way without doubt or question. But I just can't. My source of strength doesn't come from religion.

It's confusing. I like the way the Indigo Girls said it in their song, "Closer to Fine." "There's more than one answer to these questions/Pointing me in a crooked line/The less I seek my source for some definitive/The closer I am to fine." I love that song. It's just what I think about sometimes when it comes to religion, based on my experiences. I know other people think differently, and they are happy with their beliefs. That's fine too.

Anyway, for the wedding reception, we visited and booked the resort where my brother Scott had worked at one time. This inn was nestled in a picturesque background of green mountains. The resort event planner was ready to take care of all the details. We completed our tasks in Vermont, enjoying a sense of accomplishment, and continued on to Canada. I flew home and counted the days until we would be together forever. My mom and I went dress shopping, ordered invitations, and picked out a menu with the resort. My dad was giving us few budget constraints. He also loved to throw a big party.

In May, Steve flew down, and we drove my packed Vega back together. I was moving to Canada to join him in his mom's house. The immigration process was easier for me to move north of the border, so that's where we planned to begin our life together. Once again, my parents met my decision to leave the country in their classic laissez-faire style. My mom shed a tear at my departure. She told me later she shed many more once I was out of sight. I do believe I brought great joy to my mom's existence. But I was grown, and I was leaving home. My mom had planted in me all the right seeds, even though she didn't tend to the garden much, very little weeding, pruning, or additional fertilizing. I was always allowed to grow unconstrained, developing into my own form of flower. I wonder about that now, Mom, was that lack of cultivating purposeful, was it just emotional exhaustion, or was it simply neglect? Maybe Joan just believed in me that much. I don't know. There were times I felt I needed tending to. Steve fulfilled that need. He drove me away with his garden tools and his fertilizer safely placed in the trunk of my car underneath my suitcase filled with jeans and tee-shirts.

I don't know if I could have avoided interfering if my daughter told me she wanted to quit school, move to Canada, and get married at twenty years old. My mom's lack of interference resulted in my happiness and success. It could have resulted in disaster though. How can one know? Either way, when young adults make their own decisions, I'm convinced they more easily accept any consequences, whether they are positive or negative. I heard one time that parents should only interfere in their child's decision if the behavior is morally wrong or physically harmful. Moving to Canada with the love of my life was neither.

So when the big day arrived, the resort was flooded with friends and family enjoying a weekend getaway, and the Vermont magic infiltrated into the guests. There were so many pleasurable activities ready to engage anyone at any time. In fact, the day of the wedding, I climbed Deer's Leap, a great hiking trail on a nearby mountain, and I raced down the alpine slide at Pico Peak with a big group of adventuresome guests. I got back to the resort in time to primp with my friends for an hour or two before our church departure. The six o'clock wedding ceremony went perfectly, and the reception was stupendous, eating, drinking, and dancing until midnight.

Steve and I splurged on a honeymoon to Bermuda, and we celebrated my twenty-first birthday and the one year anniversary of the day we met on the island. That trip was one of many, first as a married couple, and later as a family, where walking on the beach hand in hand became an annual given. There is something mesmerizing about the smell, the sound, and the sight of that amazing horizon. Steve and I both are instantly transported to a place of harmony. Steve is always ready with his camera for gorgeous sunrise or sunset photographs. And our fondness for the local seafood completes every trip. The ocean will always have special meaning for us; it's where we began.

Upon our return home to Canada, Steve carried on with his mechanic work, and I found a job as a waitress. We moved into our rented basement apartment in a bungalow that we had been cleaning up for the last month. It wasn't much, but it was all we needed. The apartment didn't contain a kitchen per se. A laundry room was converted to a kitchen type area, housing a sink and a stove. The refrigerator had to live across the hall in the furnace room. The furnace room was also the perfect place to ferment the grape juice in big buckets that we turned into homemade wine. Bottled wine was expensive, and frugality was in my blood. I could make four meals out of one inexpensive whole chicken, baked breasts one night, barbeque legs the next, the carcass in a pot for vegetable soup the next night, and I picked the meat off the bones for chicken salad on the last night. The dining table we picked up at a garage sale was located in the hall. We had an empty living room and a bedroom complete with a bed and dresser. We were ecstatically in love and just so happy to be alone together and leave the farewells behind us forever. We made a home in our basement apartment complete with our dog, Canuck, and a new, black lab mix puppy Steve rescued. We named her Georgia.

One day, I put Canuck and Georgia out in the back yard. We had a clothesline that ran from the house to a tree at the opposite side of the yard. I figured I could throw a really long rope over the clothesline and tie the dogs to either end. Soon after tying the knots and returning to my chores, I heard Georgia squealing. I ran out to the yard and saw her hanging from the clothesline! Canuck was checking out something intently in the far corner of the lot, pulling the rope tight to dangle Georgia five feet up in the air. I guess I didn't take into consideration the differences in their weights. I held Georgia up, so she would choke no longer, and I screamed. What could I do? I wasn't strong enough to hurl her over the clothesline. Even if I could, how could I catch her on the way down the other side? Canuck would not come to me when I called, and I could see he had wrapped himself and the rope around a swing set pole. I screamed some more. My arms were getting tired. Luckily, the upstairs neighbor was home and ran out with scissors. I guess she heard my screams and looked out the back window. She cut the rope, and we laughed and cried simultaneously.

That is my favorite dumb, new bride story. I think young couples probably have lots of inexperienced, dumb stories. I am responsible for most of the ones in our marriage. When I stopped crying, I called Steve at work to tell him what happened. Repeating the ordeal just made me cry all over again. I almost killed our new dog named Georgia.

I worked at a fine restaurant Monday through Friday in what they referred to as a "Businessman's Lunch." A Greek family owned the restaurant. I asked my boss if I could work a few nights to make more money. He told me women work the lunch shift, and men work the dinner shift. I told him that was unfair and discriminatory because you make a lot more money at night. He explained in his heavy accent, "If a woman goes out for a nice dinner with her husband, and the waitress is a beautiful, young lady, her husband looks at the waitress, and the wife feels jealous. This is not good."

I responded to him, "If I go to a nice dinner with my husband, and I look at the handsome young waiter, and my husband feels jealous, what is the difference here?" He looked at me oddly. This restaurant had a way to go with the Women's Movement. I found that all the nice restaurants in the area had the same setup, so I kept waitressing during lunchtime and got a job in a clothing store at the mall a few nights a week and on weekends. Working hard was an expectation instilled in me from my parents. My mother taught me that idle time could always be spent making money somehow, and living beyond your means is bad, and saving for a rainy day is good.

After a little more than a year of Canadian living, we made the decision to head south. Real estate was more expensive in Canada, so owning a home was too far off. The prices of homes in Georgia appealed to Steve. I had quit school after leaving Georgia and wanted to return. Tuition was also cheaper in the States. Steve said he was up for the warm weather too. I'm not sure Steve's mom ever forgave me for taking away her only son. It did give her a new place to travel to, and she managed to come down at least once a year. She enjoyed the southern hospitality. It's true. As soon as you cross the Mason-Dixon line, customer service becomes as sweet as pecan pie. We continued to visit the Great White North each year as well. Steve's mom was happy for our successes although I know she missed Steve tremendously. My mom was ecstatic with my return to Georgia.

In Georgia, Steve had no trouble getting a mechanic's job. He had dirty fingernails and a certified license. I found employment at a new restaurant a young guy had started. He named it T. J. Applebee's, and that guy became quite a success story. We moved forward with our new life in the sunny South. We bought a fixer-upper and fixed it up. It was a much neglected, three bedroom, one bath, small brick ranch house, and it was the next step in the constant chain of home improvement projects that have infused our life since our marriage began. I must admit, whenever Steve puts on his old Levi's, his flannel shirt, and his work boots, my heart skips a beat. Whether he is asking me where I'd like the hole dug for a new tree we bought, or whether he is asking me to hand him a wrench while he's under the sink fixing a leak, or whether he's sanding the dining room table he's refinishing, or whether he's changing the oil in my car, I absolutely love watching and helping my handy man do something to brighten our existence. It's the best foreplay ever.

As my marriage was delightfully awakening, my parents' marriage was fading and dissolving. My mom opened up to me about the cheating that had plagued her marriage. I remember being surprised at that news. Any knowledge of that shit was buried deep at that time. While I was visiting with my dad one day after my parents' separation, we discussed that topic of infidelity. I asked him to explain his ways, why he did what he did. He was telling me about the Madonna-whore complex that he suffered from. Wives aren't sexually appealing because they are mother figures. How times have changed. Mothers have come a long way, often being referred to as MILFs today. So on that day, my father also explained to me that cheating was part of a man's makeup, and all men did it, a nice thing to say to your newly wedded daughter. I told my father that Raquel Welch could walk naked in front of Steve, and he would turn red and tell her, "No thanks, I'm in love with my wife." At that moment, my father looked at me with an expression of pity, just like I was the stupidest girl in the world. That expression was burned into my memory, ready to flash before my eyes at any moment. An irreversible severance in my relationship with my father occurred that day, and he never even picked up on it. Sad.

As a daughter of a cheating man, I had obvious issues with trust. I learned later in another psychology class that the unhealthy phenomenon of transference was occurring when I doubted my husband's ability to remain faithful based on my past experiences with my father. Steve was patient with me as I worked on internalizing what I knew to be true yet continued to doubt in moments of regression. Because Steve consistently put the needs of those he loved before his own, my belief system steadily evolved. Men do exist who avoid the sexualizing of women, whether they are the sexually deficient Madonnas, or the sexually charged MILFs. There are gentlemen who see women as human beings first, gentlemen who believe that sex is best when coupled with the one they love for life. Imagine that. And fathers should tell their daughters about these men, to look for these men. When young women hear that all men are pigs, they settle for pigs. And when fathers tell their young daughters that boys only want one thing, they are making a big mistake. Girls want boys, so the girls give the boys the one thing their daddies told them boys wanted.

I was lucky, and my marriage was thriving. We were good for each other, Steve and I. Steve was cautious and reflective. I was reckless and impulsive. That's balance, and the rubbing off on each other benefited us both. Steve showed me that keeping the wallpaper submerged in the water for the right amount of time, not half the amount of time, kept it on the wall better. He explained the purpose of preheating the oven when I burned the cookies. He showed me that leaving a neighborhood party early, before I had one more drink and fell into the Christmas tree while dancing with the dog, was a good thing. He showed me the benefits of rule following, and he provided me with some much needed boundaries. Mental health professionals would suggest emotional maturity before embarking in a lifetime relationship, but Steve guided me while I reached for my improved self. It worked.

Steve's improved self grew with my assistance as well. Steve was raised in a protected, safe, and clean environment. He experienced a home with two parents who loved each other and spent time with the kids. His parents declined the invitations to neighborhood parties in the late sixties and early seventies. They went on picnics to the lake every Saturday in the summer. A roast was in the oven every Sunday in the winter. He was awakened to the sound of a vacuum cleaner. He had to have a tidy room before he could partake in play activity.

He never got to build forts with blankets and encyclopedias. His friends didn't come over to his house to play because they might make a mess. Steve's house had rules and consequences, and conforming was the only option. His sense of stability was intact, but it was hard for him to embrace the unknown, to be spontaneous. Not making waves was a rule to live by, and risk-taking behavior was not encouraged. Because perfection was sought after, Steve learned to question his confidence. "If you are going to do something, then do it right" is really very limiting. I like "If you can walk you can dance; if you can talk you can sing" better. When Steve found the note in his desk from his mommy after a PTA meeting, it said, "I like your classroom. Some of your penmanship could be a little neater, Stephen. Love, Mommy." My mom's note to me after PTA nights would just say everything was wonderful, and I was wonderful. We had different expectations, eh?

So I helped Steve learn how to loosen up and take life less seriously. I showed him that walking outside in your slippers wouldn't hurt a thing. Dishes in the sink could wait until morning. I convinced him that dressing like a woman for our neighborhood Halloween party would be fun. I showed him how to apply mascara and put on pantyhose. He accepted the plan to drive along the North Carolina Outer Banks on vacation without any hotel reservations, to be flexible with the itinerary. One never knows what unexpected treasure might be found. We admired and didn't discount each other's outlook on life. I am always amazed by his integrity and preparedness. I asked him recently to name one thing he loved about me. He replied, "You aren't afraid of anything."

We are still deeply in love, probably more so, over twenty-five years later. The empty nest has allowed us to revisit some of those liberated habits of youth, and we both find the situation quite enjoyable. Steve still bends over and unties his tennis shoes before he removes them. He wouldn't think about drinking straight from the milk jug in the fridge. I can steal a swig when no one is looking, and I put my toe to my heel, dig in, and fling every time I remove my tied up tennis shoes. On our roller coaster ride of life, Steve always makes sure my lap belt is securely fastened, and I tell him to throw his arms up in the air on the big hills.

Chapter 10   The Madness

With Joan residing at Country Gardens, we felt relieved, and our load eased. She was close and safe, meals were being prepared for her, her medication was being properly dispensed, and she still enjoyed a sense of autonomy. It was almost blissful. We noticed upon her arrival that she looked in better shape than many of the other residents. Her physical activity level was beyond the capabilities of every resident. Her mental capacity was at par with most. This allowed Joan to be the helper when it was time to pass out supplies for a craft activity. When the magician came to put on a show, Joan was up in a flash to be the audience participant. It was great, and the nursing aides who worked at Country Gardens loved Joan's enthusiasm.

Joan befriended the lady across the hall, Charlotte. Charlotte had that beautiful, sophisticated, Old South drawl. Joan and Charlotte would stroll around the perimeter of the building together. They sat next to each other at the same dining table. I joined that table about once a week for dinner. Charlotte asked me what I did, and I told her I was a counselor at a high school. She replied, "I taught elementary school for many years. I never had a bad student in my classroom, just mischievous students." I loved Charlotte for that statement alone. We would share teaching stories as we both taught the fourth grade for some years. The problem was the next week, when I'd sit down to dinner, Charlotte would turn to me and ask, "Hello there, and what do you do?"

Many of the residents were in some state of dementia, Alzheimer's, I suppose. Senility is what they used to call it. The label made no difference. They varied in severity, but the disparity was also evident in the rate of deterioration. Edith met us at the door the day we arrived. She was obviously suffering from confusion, but she was a joyous soul. About a year later, the day I removed Mom's final belongings from her room, Edith met me at the door with the exact same personality, expression, and conversation she shared with us our first day at Country Gardens. In that same amount of time, Joan went from pretty good functioning to non-functioning.

There were very few men at the facility, three most of the time. Two were named Ned, and one was named Saul. We named them speckled head Ned, wheel chair Ned, and Pall Mall Saul. Saul smoked on his patio. It took a while to get used to witnessing the interactions in an assisted living residence. One day, early on in Joan's stay, speckled head Ned asked an aide why there were balloons in the dining room. She bellowed forcefully right in his ear, "It's Saul's birthday!" Steve and I were rather taken aback at the volume level of her voice, and we thought it was rather rude of her to yell so loudly directly into the old man's ear.

Speckled head Ned just looked at her and asked, "What?" Steve and I snickered together at our naivety.

Wheelchair Ned lived in the room at the end of the hall right next to Mom's room. He fell one night and cut his head badly. He died a few days later in the hospital. There were blood stains on the carpet outside of his door at the end of the hall. Attempts were made to remove the stains to no avail. Every time Steve visited Joan, while approaching her door, he would look at those stains and ask me, "When are they going to replace that carpet?"

Mom became accustomed to her new surroundings, but she unfortunately continued to mentally deteriorate at a fast pace. It was happening too quickly, and we so wanted to enjoy this new living arrangement for a while. It was much more manageable than the last year or so visiting her in her old home. I would arrive at Country Gardens each weekday around three thirty, right after work. Mom and I would go for a walk around the building and then sit in her room. We tried to carry on small conversations. She wanted to talk about her divorce sometimes. "I shouldn't have divorced your father. I broke up a family." I'd reassure her that we were all fine and that the decision was exactly what she wanted to do at that point in her life. I forgot sometimes and talked to her like she understood rational thoughts. She responded with, "Do you think he'd take me back?" She had no idea that Dad had been married to Doris for twenty years.

I was puzzled by Joan's statement and question. She had waited a long time and had struggled with her decision to divorce my dad. Once it was over, she always seemed content with her choice. She didn't bring it up much and seemed very satisfied in her independent life. But I guess divorce is a sad satisfaction, probably filled with mourning what could have been, or what should have been. Were her thoughts that day a true regret, or were they due to a diseased and misfiring brain? Our hidden thoughts rarely emerge while we're in complete control. My guess is by losing control, she spoke her truth. But as her disease progressed, many of her thoughts were nonsensical. It was probably wrong to interpret meanings to her words. I don't know.

Once, while in the midst of my troubled youth, my parents picked me up at a neighborhood bar and brought me home. My boyfriend called them as he was worried about my drunken state. Mom, Dad, and I sat at the kitchen table, and I slurred out my knowledge of Dad's affairs. It must have been that earlier diary reading escaping from its hiding place. It waited until I was out of control. I don't remember much about that night, but I do remember my parents' shocked facial expressions as their secret was revealed through my slurs. None of us ever brought that night up again. I bet they thought I was too drunk to remember the conversation. I guess I wasn't. That knowledge retreated back to its deep hiding place that night in my sleep. Secrets can go into remission. I can't even recall now at what point in my life the memory from that dysfunctional night felt safe enough to emerge and live in the open. Weird.

So anyway, I tried to take Joan out once and a while for a change of scenery. We walked to a local art festival in the historic downtown area about one mile away from County Gardens one warm autumn day. Art was one of Joan's favorite pastimes, both the creating and the appreciating. She walked by the booths like she was walking by blank space. Joan showed no interest in anything we saw. I kept trying to pull her in saying, "Look Mom, look at this unusual use of stained glass. Isn't it beautiful?" She just glanced at the work of art and kept walking. It was so strange for me. This behavior was so unlike Mom. Something that brought her such joy in the past no longer initiated any kind of reaction. That's just another example of the shittiness of the disease. We walked back to her apartment in silence. She never mentioned a word to me or to anyone about her day at the art festival. The old Joan would have raved about it for weeks.

We looked at the mail she received, and I'd read it to her. She acquired lots of mail in the beginning. I had written a letter and sent it to all her friends, near and far, when Joan entered Country Gardens. I informed them of her inability to remain on her own, the need for assisted living, and I described her new, pleasant surroundings. I included her change of address and new phone number. Most had recognized the troubles in Joan, and this news did not come as a surprise.

I asked her to read the mail to me periodically. I was amazed as I watched her reading skills regress in the opposite sequence reading skills were typically learned. She would read easy words and fumble over longer, more difficult words. Each month would get worse. Her comprehension went from some to none while she lived in her apartment at Country Gardens. When she was finding it difficult to write a note to a friend, we moved to dictation, just like a preschooler. Eventually, by the end, she lost the ability to write her own name. It was peculiar for me, watching the regression. I had spent many years teaching in elementary schools observing children moving forward in reading fluency, comprehension, and writing skills.

The TV in Joan's room was useless to her. Sometimes at four o'clock, I'd turn on her television to watch Oprah. She would sit and look at me or pace around her room. She had no interest in any topic whatsoever. I'd leave at five when it was time for her dinner, walking her to her table on my way out the door. I'd get home a little before Steve got home from work. It was a doable routine; my own children were grown and out of the house. I remember reading something about the difficulties of those who had the job of caring for their children and their parents at the same time. The sandwich generation, it was called. I was thankful I didn't fall into that category. I was able to give my mom the full attention she needed.

Scott stopped to visit Mom in the evening on his way home from work. He continued to sit at her kitchen table, hold her hand, and just be. He brought her peace. He also bought all her favorites, Andes Candies, jars of grapefruit sections, yogurt, and ginger ale, which kept her little dorm room fridge well-stocked. On my visits, I continued to pick up the dirty tissues scattered about, empty her trash, take home her laundry, and remind her to get in the shower. Again, she would say I was scolding her when I told her to stop sticking her used panty liners to the bathroom hand railings. This had become some new bizarre habit, going through five a day, lining them up in a neat row on the hand railings, and not disposing of them properly. I couldn't stand it. "Mom, panty liners are not to be seen! Throw them away after you use them! Flush them down the toilet, or put them in the garbage! Just stop sticking them to the bathroom hand rails!" Some things didn't change with the new living arrangement.

She was going to the bathroom a lot, so I took her to her doctor. They could find nothing wrong, no infection, no abnormal test results. She complained about something in her eye one day, and I could not help her no matter how many drops I put in her eye, so I took her to the eye doctor. They could find nothing in her eye to cause irritation. They did suggest we come back for a complete eye exam because they noticed some cataracts that were forming. About this time, I had also received reminders from her dentist that it was time for a cleaning. All her official mail was being delivered to my house since she moved to Country Gardens. I had a day off from work coming up, so I thought about making an eye appointment in the morning and a dental appointment in the afternoon. We could go out for lunch in between. It would be like old times.

Scott and I had a conversation about her doctor appointments. Our family had never been quick to visit doctors. As kids, our parents gave us juice and put us to bed rather than run to the doctor. My dad explained to me how fevers were actually trying to kill the invading virus or bacteria; fevers were beneficial. He was on the anti antibiotic bandwagon before it was popular. He told me I was equipped with antibodies to fight off infection and taking an antibiotic would just weaken my own immune system by killing my good bacteria. So it was natural for both Scott and I to question how many doctor's visits were really necessary for Mom. She was going to the neurologist every four months. She had always visited the eye doctor and dentist regularly. And of course, I had just taken her to the eye doctor and general practice doctor for her phantom problems. Truthfully, she didn't even wear her glasses anymore. At first, it was because she could never find them. Then, it was because she didn't know what they were for. Could I postpone these checkups a little more? I even contemplated skipping them. She became so confused at her appointments. Scott thought we should let her be. I consulted with Lea Anne about the situation, seeing as she was in the dental field. She believed strongly about continuing all of Joan's care. I felt so guilty about questioning the need for maintenance care. I was flirting with selfishness. So I made the appointments.

I picked up Mom the morning of our appointments. After repeating to her where we were going the entire car ride to the eye doctor, we finally arrived. She enjoyed the attention from the doctor, and I helped her answer questions she didn't understand. They dilated her pupils and found evidence of some early macular degeneration and some small cataract development. We discussed treatment options. But after the doctor observed the confused state of Joan, he also questioned the need to follow through with interventions. Joan put on quite a show. She freaked out over the side effects of the dilation procedure. She was screaming at the doctor, "I can't see! I could see before I came to this office, and I can't now!" I tried to explain the process to her, how she would recover soon. I tried to get her to remember that she had had her pupils dilated many times before at the eye doctor. But she would have none of it. "I have never been blind before. They made me blind! I can't see!" The patients in the waiting room gave me looks of compassion and understanding as I escorted my mom out of the office, all the while listening to her yell, "I can't see! I can't see! I could see when I got here! They have blinded me! I'm blind, I tell you!"

We didn't go to lunch, obviously. I took her to my house and helped her lie down on the couch. I figured maybe she would fall asleep and wake up with the effects of the dilation drops gone. She didn't fall asleep, but she rested long enough to recover. I made lunch for us, and she seemed to forget that anything occurred. She just started acting like Joan from Country Gardens again, no mention of the morning eye exam. We set off for the dentist. It was just a cleaning. What could possibly go wrong?

I played the car radio a little louder than usual on the way to the dentist appointment to avoid answering the question about where we were going over and over. We went into the office, and everyone was happy to see Joan. She had been going to the same dentist for thirty years. They took her back to the examining room. I read magazines in the waiting room. When she returned, the hygienist explained to me that Mom had said her bottom tooth was sharp. The dentist tried to smooth it out, but Mom was not satisfied. The dentist couldn't feel any sharpness, but Mom could. I told them not to worry. They gave me that familiar look. We left the dentist office with waiting room patients staring again in those compassionate expressions. Joan was screaming, "What did they do to me? My bottom tooth is as sharp as a razor! It's cutting my tongue! It's so sharp, I'm telling you! My tooth is cutting my tongue to pieces! My tongue is bleeding! It hurts! I'll never come here again!"

Again, I turned up my radio on the way home to drown out the complaining. But by the time we got back to her place, she had settled down. By supper all was forgotten, forgotten by Joan, but not by me. The day was very unnerving, but what choice did I have? I guess I just needed to be more prepared next time. She caught me off guard that day. What was I thinking, like old times? Because I always had summers free, those days were easily spent with Joan whenever necessary. Through the years, we enjoyed days like that together, lunching, shopping, sightseeing, and following through with her appointments. Not anymore, just taking her to the store to get some cough drops or panty liners, two items she was paranoid about running out of, was now a nightmare.

I guess another goodbye was appropriate at that moment, a goodbye to logical practices. Everyday activities, not the intellectual ones, the mundane ones, were becoming impossible. When your parent has Alzheimer's, life becomes a series of goodbyes, the first one sad and each subsequent one just as sad. The Joan we knew and loved kept disappearing one chunk at a time. There was nothing anyone could do about it.

Joan was really losing her mind. Her confusion was turning into madness, showing up infrequently at first and more often as time went on. Steve and I, and Bonnie and Lee planned a trip to Canada to attend the wedding of Steve's nephew. We decided that we could fly to Buffalo and rent a car to complete the trip to Ontario. We could take Joan with us, leave her in Buffalo, and let her have a visit with her two brothers and their families. We realized that this might be the last time she could visit with her Buffalo family. They, too, obviously noticed the changes in Joan over the last couple of years. She always enjoyed trips to her home state, and Scott had accompanied her more than once over the past few years when traveling alone was becoming more difficult. Joan's niece, our cousin Linda, was a nurse and could put Joan up for the weekend.

When we sat down on the plane, preparing for flight, mom leaned over to me and whispered, "We're going to crash, but I'm a survivor." I leaned over the aisle to repeat her comments to Steve. He passed them on to the kids like a game of telephone. When we arrived in

Buffalo, she didn't respond at first. This surprised us as Joan talked about Buffalo all the time. A trip to Buffalo meant excitement and satisfaction. Half way to her brother George's house, while riding in the rental car, she saw a sign and yelled out, "Grand Island? We're in Buffalo? Yippee!"

We settled her in and went on our way to the wedding in Ontario. I called Linda and got updates. Linda was an awesome lady and handled Joan beautifully. Mom went to a cook out and spent time with her Buffalo family. Even though Mom wasn't her old self, she enjoyed the trip. I found that people were generally understanding in her presence. Supportive glances and encouraging expressions were common from strangers. I hoped Linda had similar experiences as she entertained Joan. We picked her up again at the end of the weekend and boarded the plane headed to Atlanta.

We sat down in the same configuration, Mom and I on one side, and Steve, Bonnie, and Lee on the other side of the aisle. As soon as we were settled, Mom whispered to me, "That's George and that's Linda," pointing to the two people sitting in front of us. She kept telling me George and Linda were in front of us. The two heads were those of an elderly man and a dark, curly haired woman, very similar to the backs of George and Linda's heads. I tried to explain that she had just said good-bye to them, and yes, they had a lovely visit, but now we were on our way home. George and Linda were back in Buffalo. She kept on. She started reaching over the back of the seats in front of us trying to pat the heads of "George and Linda." I was grabbing at her hand but missed eventually. The woman in front of us turned around, and I explained that my mom was confused and thought she knew her. I apologized. Mom persisted. "I'm telling you, that's George, and that's Linda." She was saying this more loudly each time. My telling her that it wasn't George and Linda had no impact. When the "fasten your seat belt" light went out, I unbuckled us both and walked Mom into the aisle to get a good look at the couple in front of us. Mom looked at them and then looked at me and said, "You're right."

Steve and the kids were trying not to laugh. It usually starts out funny, those moments of madness. Then, when everything calms down and you have time to process the events that occur, you find yourself fighting back tears, not laughter.

Bonnie told me she saw Grandma talking to herself in the mirror at Christmas time. By January, Joan's nonsense talk was becoming serious. She told me Country Gardens had run out of food, and they had nothing to eat. She told the nursing aides that she was moving to Buffalo to live with Linda. She told Mark on the phone that I was on my way to pick her up to take her to the hospital when I wasn't. She called up my mother in law in Canada and told her that I was in the hospital. Her thoughts were jumbled, her statements, fiction. She started calling me numerous times a day and leaving messages on my answering machine that just made no sense. She'd start by asking if I was there, then when she'd get no response, she'd just talk to me like I was on the phone with her. Sometimes, she left messages that were conversations she had with herself. She would alternate between a regular speaking voice, a yelling voice, and a scary, whisper voice. "Candy, are you there? Candy? It's Saturday. No, no, it's Sunday. She said I should shower today. No, it's Saturday. It's dark now. Candy should be home. She shouldn't be out this late. IT'S DARK OUT! Alright, it's Sunday. Yes, it's Sunday." Then, she'd hang up.

Nothing was as bizarre as her fearful stories concerning Scott though. I arrived at her place one day, and she was crying. "What's wrong, Mom?" I asked.

"Scotty. He doesn't have a father." She replied.

"Sure he does, Mom, the same father I have, Harry. We both saw him over Christmas time."

"Well, Scotty doesn't have a wife."

"Sure he does, Mom. He's happily married to Diana. They live close by."

"Well, Scotty doesn't have a job."

"Mom, he goes to work every day. He stops here after work often."

The next day followed a similar pattern. I found her distraught. "Scotty doesn't have a driver's license or a car."

I explained, "Yes, he does Mom. He drives over here many nights to visit you in his car. He's coming to visit you tonight in his car."

Then she started the new, scary whisper voice. "He is in jail, Candy. He was sleeping in the building across the street. He stole a car. Someone called the police. He stole a car. I just found out."

I just looked at her. There was no point in arguing. We went for a walk, and she slowly returned to her form of normal, not the definition of normal most would use. Scott and I maintained our daily phone conversations keeping each other up to date with Mom stories throughout her entire stay at Country Gardens, just like when she lived alone. There was always something to touch base about. I phoned him this particular afternoon to tell him about what Mom was saying. After he visited her, he came by our house to talk about Mom. We opened a beer, started a conversation about the crazy mother we shared, and the phone rang. It was Mom. She was yelling, "Turn on the news! Scotty is on the news. He stole a car. He just stole a car! He's on the news. Turn on your TV right now, Candy!"

The day we took the phone out of her room was the day she called Mark to inform him that Scott was dead. It was uncomfortable letting Scott know about this most recent madness talk. She was turning into a freak. We were entering the world of delusion.

It's hard to explain my feelings at this point. Conflicted is a good term. This woman was my mother. This woman was not my mother. I had to care deeply for this person. I had to remove myself emotionally from this person. I was weakened by her exorbitant needs even though I was somewhat disturbingly intrigued by her strange talk and thought processes. I was thankful I had so many supportive people around me with whom to share this conflicting journey. Her disease was the topic of many conversations. My cousin and I compared the physical difficulties her dad was experiencing with the intellectual difficulties my mom was experiencing. Linda thought losing your mind was more difficult than losing your body. I thought for the rest of the family, perhaps, but for the patient, I don't know. Mom was unaware of her plight, my uncle was frustratingly aware of his physical disabilities.

We knew Mom was way beyond her Aricept prescription. When she had a check up with the neurologist, he just upped the dosage when we talked about some of her newer symptoms. He added Namenda as well, a drug for more advanced stages of Alzheimer's.

Honestly, I questioned the effectiveness of the medication used for her illness. I questioned the benefits of the neurologist himself. He offered little assistance, little advice. He was good for an exam and a prescription, neither of which helped much. On one of her visits to his office, she became silly on the exam table. The doctor was asking her to touch her nose and then touch his finger. He made his finger a moving target and asked her to keep touching her nose and then touch his finger. He was checking on coordination, I presume. She thought it was a funny assignment, so she stuck her thumbs in her ears, stuck her fingers out like moose antlers, and wiggled her fingers at him. She used to make that gesture whenever she felt Steve was going overboard with the camera shots in her direction. She was always finding opportunities for silliness. My mother taught me to find humor in, or to bring humor to, every corner of life as often as possible. That day, I was thankful to see she had not lost this humor completely and that a little of Joan was still in there. I was laughing with her, but the doctor wasn't amused. His bedside manner left much to be desired.

At the last appointment she participated in with this neurologist, she was very frustrated. The same mini mental exam was given, but this time, she couldn't answer many questions. She couldn't perform many tasks. She was mad that they didn't ask her the question she knew the answer to, the question and answer set she had been practicing daily. She practiced in the car on the way to the doctor's office. When the doctor failed to ask her the information she wanted to share, she insisted on telling him anyway as we were walking down the hall toward the exit. "I have three children. Scott was born in

1951. Mark was born in 1954, and Candy was born in 1961." She was so proud of herself for remembering those important facts. It was her most valuable and treasured information. It was one of the last bits of sanity she had left. I was smiling through my tears as I listened to the pride in her voice as she recited her precious knowledge to the uninterested doctor.

Scott and I knew she was getting close to being beyond what an assisted living facility could handle, but we didn't want to face the prospect of change so soon. With the house sale work still fresh in my memory, I just yearned for a span of time without too many hassles. It felt like I just got her settled, all of us in a routine. I wasn't ready for another move. Just like we did at the final stages of her independence at her house, we reacted with providing Joan more face time and more interventions. We tried to make Mom the perfect resident. We kept her apartment and her things neat. We visited as much as we could to give them a break. We didn't want her to be a burden, and we didn't want her caregivers to decide she could no longer stay in her comfortable apartment. The phone calls from Country Gardens were increasing. "Joan has broken the door knob again. She won't stop messing with it because she can't figure out how to lock or unlock the door. Joan won't eat. Joan won't take her medicine." Each time the phone rang, I'd panic. We didn't know what was coming next. No one was telling us what to do. I probably should have reached out to some Alzheimer's organization for some guidance. But by this point, I never had the time to surf the web for information or go to support group sessions. I spent my time gathering the information first hand. It just went so fast. She wasn't the same Joan that entered the Country

Gardens doors just five months earlier. She didn't participate in many daily activities anymore. The only thing that made Joan perk up lately, the only activity she would join in, was the visits from the children. A local private school that was close by came to visit the old folks periodically, and children always made Joan happy.

Throughout her life, Joan delighted in children. "Look at that beautiful child," she verbalized on many occasions. Most of all, she loved to make them smile. She always knelt down to connect to the child's eye level and present herself as an equal to any child she encountered. I must credit her example, as well as the births of my two children, for my decision to spend my life surrounded by wee ones, both my own kids and my borrowed kids, the students.

Chapter 11 The Children

Very early in my marriage I wanted to become pregnant. I guess I wanted a baby, so I could experience and embrace the happy, healthy, and precious family life I so desired. I don't think I analyzed my reasons back then; I only knew I wanted a baby. Marrying a man that was the opposite of my father was only the first step in my healing process. Steve was excited about becoming a Daddy too. We had our first little house all set, and we were successful at conception right away. Again, mental health professionals would probably say we were too young and not financially stable enough. And I did receive more than one discriminatory glance or comment at being such a young mom. It was becoming in vogue to postpone parenthood at that time. Many people believed that young parents equaled inadequate parents. But parenthood was good for us, and those people were so wrong. We were good at it. My life found purpose and direction. The first baby and then baby number two were a perfect fit. My mom was thrilled for us. She loved coming over to our home and holding our babies.

Bonnie and Lee were beautiful babies, both of them easy-going and happy. The love Mommy and Daddy experienced upon their arrivals was unbelievable. First time parents are often unprepared for the wonderment and love that flood into their lives when they see their baby for the first time. I always ask new moms or dads that question. "You didn't know you could love someone so much, did you?" The realization that you can feel that way again is also overwhelming. "You didn't think you could love another baby as much as you did the first one, did you?" That's something I've said to second time parents. Baby love is infinite.

Bonnie arrived first. We loved and cherished our new little girl. I stayed home and nursed, sang to, and rocked my new baby. Steve participated in every aspect of taking care of her. I hadn't returned to college yet, not knowing in which direction to head. After spending a short amount of time with Bonnie, the answer became clear. I wanted to major in Early Childhood Education. I was amazed and hungry for knowledge at every stage in her development.

When she was one, I started back at Georgia State University. I sat in the front row and probably annoyed the younger students. I savored everything about my classes and ruined the curve. I continued to waitress Friday night and Sunday brunch each week to earn our spending money. That gave Steve some time alone with Bonnie. He did different stuff with her like packing a picnic lunch and going to a small, local airfield to watch the planes take off and land.

Baby Lee came two and a half years later. I put my studies on hold for a year, so I could nurse, sing to, and rock this new baby too. We also moved into a brand new neighborhood in a brand new house with two bathrooms while I was pregnant, so we were busy painting, wallpapering, and feathering a new nest. Our home improvement projects on the first fixer upper proved to be lucrative. I made homemade baby food and shopped for baby clothes at the end of each season to save us money.

When Lee was one, the three of us hiked back to Georgia State. They provided a child development day care center for students and faculty to utilize. During the lunch break, I sat in the observation rooms and ate my bagged sandwich, watching my kids through one-way glass, while most of my classmates went to the student center to eat their cafeteria lunches and watch Soaps. At home, I tried out Piaget's experiments in cognitive development on my two children. Fascinating.

It took seven years from the time I started back, twelve years after I finished high school, but I graduated Magna Cum Laude with my Early Childhood Education degree at the age of twenty-nine. Steve was so proud of me. So was my mom, and she forgave me for not wearing a cap and gown before a wedding gown. I started teaching at the neighborhood elementary school when Bonnie was in second grade and Lee was in preschool. Steve's elite Canadian training and knowledge in the automotive field and the fact that he believed in going to work every day and arriving on time brought him career advancement. He moved from mechanic to service manager to store manager within the Goodyear Company. We didn't have high salaries, but we could afford to live comfortably with our three-bedroom ranch house and two cars. The two parent, two kid, cat and dog family even enjoyed an adventurous family vacation each year.

Our journey resembled most, North and South, calm and stormy. Looking for the wonder and finding the love was the best road map. The kids were the main attraction. Just paying attention along the way to kids' thought processes always amazed and entertained me, the constant job of dealing with a state of disequilibrium and striving for a state of equilibrium, as Piaget put it. For example, Bonnie loved Frosty the Snowman. She watched that video often during the holiday season the year she was two. That year we also enjoyed a rare, substantial snowfall in Georgia. Bonnie and I were up early making a snowman in the front yard. Steve was busy with the video recorder, capturing our milestones as usual. The minute we put the finishing touches on our happy snowman face and took a step back to admire our work, Bonnie said, "Talk now. Talk snowman, talk." The Frosty story was her only experience with a snowman, so why wouldn't she think this one would come to life?

We believed in telling the kids at an early age, when they started asking questions, the truth about sex. We listened to the experts' advice, just answering the questions they had, only getting into areas that were age appropriate. When the topic arose about sex being a pleasurable part of life for couples that were in love, Lee shrieked, "You mean you did that more than twice?" Guiding your kids through the confusing world and noticing how they figure it all out was too much fun.

Bonnie's personality was tailored from Steve, his genes completely. She wanted to follow the rules from day one. Lee's personality was the opposite. Beginning about the time he turned one year old, he challenged order at every opportunity, more like my side of the family. I learned in one psychology class about the nature versus nurture argument. I was constantly adjusting my opinion upon which carried the higher percentage of importance. Were we a blank slate at birth, or did we come pre-wired for life? I agreed with the majority of experts, figuring it was probably fifty-fifty. I knew I had a real scientific experiment at home. I was the female role model for a daughter born with the reflective temperament of her father. Steve was the male role model for a son born with the impulsive temperament of his mother. It was classic nature vs. nurture stuff.

When Bonnie started kindergarten, she was introduced to the Friday ice cream treat routine. On her first decision-making day, she picked out a Fudgsicle. She came home all excited about the yumminess of the Fudgsicle. She said, "They have lots of ice creams to pick from, but my Fudgsicle was so good, I'm going to get that one every Friday!"

When Lee started kindergarten and was introduced to the Friday ice cream treat routine, he had a different approach. He picked out an ice cream sandwich. He came home all excited about the yumminess of the ice cream sandwich. He said, "They have lots of different ice cream, and I'm going to try every one of them until I've tried them all!" The theme of their subsequent early life encounters is summed up in that story: safety vs. risk, Steve vs. Candy.

Bonnie was opening her stocking one Christmas morning. "A tooth brush! Just what I always wanted!" she exclaimed. She was always trying to please us. The first time she was old enough to go over to a friend's house to play, she called home after about an hour. She wanted permission to eat a cookie. We had to push her sometimes to take a risk. She'll probably never forgive us for making her go down the class four rapids on a white water river rafting trip. It was a family venture, and we weren't going to let her get out of that raft and miss the excitement. She survived, but she didn't smile when it was over.

Bonnie sailed through childhood with many friends and few troubles. She was a teacher's pet and a good student. She was beautiful inside and out. She loved to sing and dance to her Raffi tapes. She loved her animals. We all took pleasure in the typical family pets, a golden retriever named Raji and a tabby cat named Tara, but none more than Bonnie. Bonnie collected critters whenever the opportunity arose. She brought a roly-poly bug in a match box to her seventh grade desk, just to keep and take care of while at school. She was creative, always making crafty treasures out of household items while sitting on the floor in her bedroom. She appreciated and recognized beauty all around her. Once, she rescued plastic forks from the trash after a birthday party. I found them under her dresser. She told me the colors were too pretty to throw away. She made wise decisions and was a breeze to raise.

I told her only once that she let me down. She came home from ninth grade one day with information about the upcoming Miss Freshman pageant. I cried out, "What have I done wrong? How could I have raised a daughter who wants to be in a beauty pageant! I hate beauty pageants!" She knew I was kidding, but not kidding either. We actually went right over to Grandma Joan's house and dug up this beautiful, iridescent, plum colored gown Grandma had worn to a formal as a young woman. It fit Bonnie perfectly, and Bonnie looked stunning in it. My mom and I thought she should have won that stupid pageant. A cheerleader won. Bonnie enjoyed participating in the pageant, but thankfully, it was her last. Her eager-to-please personality sometimes worried me that the world might eat her up. I made it a point to constantly encourage and groom her independence, just as my mom had done for me.

Lee sat at the dinner table one night when he was only five and stated, "Three and a half chickens were killed for this meal." There were seven chicken legs on the plate in the center of the table. He often made us shake our heads and laugh with his unusual observations of life. He wandered off by himself wherever we went, be it the backyard, the airport, the beach, or Disney World. He never thought about getting permission to explore. Steve and I were panic-stricken parents more than once. We had to squelch his uncontrollable enthusiasm for adventure at times. He had broken his arm at preschool when he was four. While attending a hot air balloon festival on vacation shortly after the cast was put on, Lee made another trip to the emergency room. Three stitches were put on the bridge of his nose due to a fall. We carried on with our vacation to the beach, the battered looking Lee in tow, and checked into the hotel. Before we could put the suitcases down, there was Lee, jumping from one double bed to the other with his arm in a cast and three fresh stitches in his head. I screamed at him.

Lee didn't sail through childhood. He struggled with friendships and authority. He had the unsatisfactory check-mark in "shows self-control" on every report card all through elementary school. He suffered from migraines and meltdowns. He loved spending most of his time with video games and Legos. He memorized the multiplication tables in a day or two by staring at the poster on his third grade classroom wall. The bullies picked on him in seventh grade. He fought back one day in the school bathroom and got suspended. He learned most things the hard way and was a challenge to raise.

Steve and I worked relentlessly with Lee. He was an impulsive, determined, and sensitive little boy who resisted change or uncertainty. Some of these qualities are often valued in adults, but not in children. People don't smile much at kids like Lee. Call it Attention Deficit/ Hyperactivity Disorder or mild Asperger's Syndrome or just plain annoying. Dealing with his personality type was difficult for most people. We even refrained from leaving Lee with Grandma or other family members very often so as to avoid conflict. There was no quick fix. I read a number of books with titles like *The Spirited Child* or *The Explosive Child* to give me knowledge and strength. We did everything we could do to provide him with positive experiences to try and keep his self esteem intact. Sticker charts decorated his bedroom door. Sometimes, we were out of patience and handled him poorly. I told him the truth. Childhood wasn't the best part of everyone's life, and we would help him get through it. I assured him regularly that he was going to make a fine young man one day. Scott told me once that the child you are is not the adult you become. I banked on that statement.

The results are in now that our children are grown. The fifty-fifty theory stands. Bonnie has not let go of her conformity completely, but my attempts at challenging her cautious character were successful. She is a confident and independent young woman. When she walks in a room, she has a way of making it become brighter. Little kids and old folks are drawn to Bonnie; they recognize her virtue somehow. Lee still treasures nonconformity, but I see Steve's calm presence in him more and more each day. He is responsible, and he is a gentleman. He still baffles me with his unusual way of seeing things. He was in need of a haircut after a stint with very long, shaggy-headed college growth. With my scissors in hand, I asked him how he wanted his hair cut. He said, "All the same length." I asked him if he really wanted it straight across his shoulders, or would he like it better layered. He explained that hair cut all the same length would in fact be layered. Hair all cut to the shoulder would be hair cut in different lengths. He's right.

The wondrous journey was not void of the occasional "Watch for Falling Rock" signs. A moment of resentment from my own childhood caught me off guard when Bonnie was thirteen years old. I studied her innocence at that age, so prevalent, and clearly saw the parents' role of protection. It hurt and angered me to think my parents were so amiss on that front. I cried a few tears for the vulnerable thirteen-year-old Candy standing on the kitchen chair to reach the liquor cabinet. I played the song, "Objects in the Rearview Mirror May Appear Closer than They Are" by Meatloaf really loud. Steve and I had numerous conversations with both the kids about alcohol, drugs, and drinking and driving when it was appropriate. It wasn't that hard to set boundaries that kept them as safe as possible. It was easy for me to pay attention to the needs of my young daughter. It was easy to encourage open communication with her as she developed from child to young woman.

It helped that Steve and I worked hard at keeping our relationship with each other strong too. We believed in putting the kids to bed early to have time for each other at night. For years, we had the routine of reading to Bonnie and Lee at bedtime. I'd start with Bonnie, and Steve started with Lee. Their rooms were right next to each other. After we finished our story, the kids would yell,

"We're done!" Then, we switched places and each read a book to the other child. No matter what was going on at the evening hour or who was visiting our house, we never missed the bedtime story routine. That practice also cast us into a nice frame of mind to enjoy the evening with each other.

Steve was such a good dad, and I was so happy for my kids. Once or twice, while I watched Steve interact with his children, I fell to a melancholy place from my past, the rocks again. I wondered how it would feel to grow up with such a sense of family, to grow up with a dad that put the kids first and was always there. But most of the time, I relished in the fact that Steve was a family man, and I experienced great joy watching him with the kids. He put their towels in the dryer to warm them while they were finishing up in the tub on cold nights. He ate two Happy Meals at McDonalds with the guys from work at lunch on Fridays, so he could bring the toys home to his kids. He made our big, special Daddy Breakfast every Sunday morning. The father of my children was present, and that was a beautiful thing.

We spent Sundays together as a family, usually choosing an outdoor event where we all could explore and enjoy nature. We didn't go to church. If a G od looked down at the four of us together, experiencing the splendid world around us, how could there be an objection? When they were little, Bonnie and Lee did go to church with Grandma sometimes. When they were a little older, we encouraged the kids to go to church with their friends when they were invited. Bonnie went to the Baptist Church with her friend Lisa a few times. Lee went to the Mormon Church with his friend Joshua a few times. But when the Baptist youth group started knocking on our door, asking for Bonnie, and telling her she was going to hell because she wasn't saved, I stepped in. I asked them to leave and not come back. Bonnie and I had a long talk about beliefs. I'm sure my bias emerged. It was uncomfortable at times for the kids as we were raising our children in the South, the Bible Belt. They were always asked, "What church do ya'll go to?" Judgment flourished when the answer was given. Bonnie still hung out with all the girls wearing their WWJD bracelets, but she became armed with a variety of contrasting philosophies. Bonnie played soccer with a girl named Mary from a zealot family. The whole family wore a rainbow of WWJD bracelets at all times. When Mary was playing soccer, her mom was screaming from the stands at the referees, the coach, and the opposing team. She was screaming unbecoming phrases. It wasn't really what Jesus would do. I wanted to tell her that so bad.

Steve and I did try to educate the kids in our own way on Christianity. We watched the movie *Jesus Christ Superstar* together. I loved that sound track. Sometimes, I wanted to try the Unitarian Church or something like that. I thought maybe I was not doing my job when my kids didn't attend regular religious services. Steve never second guessed our decision. He was comfortable with his non-believer status. He was the most caring, honest, selfless, good hearted man I knew. So how could I oppose? He taught "Christian" values through example. Many "Christians" would have been surprised to discover his views. We didn't talk much about them in public. Intolerance thrived.

We went to a Passion Play one Easter when the kids were about ten and eight. A fellow teacher had given me tickets because she was singing a solo in the show. After the story of Jesus was beautifully performed, a new set appeared on the stage with a modern day dinner party already in progress. A member of the dinner party, Jenn, clutched her chest and dropped dead from a heart attack right before dessert. Jesus appeared at the party in his white gown and clipboard, flanked on either sided by a beautiful, blonde, female angel. He told the family the bad news. Jenn was not saved, and therefore, was not going to heaven. She wasn't on his list. The family pleaded with Jesus. They told him she was a good person, a doctor who saved lives. She followed rules and was kind to everyone. Jesus just shook his head and pointed to his clipboard. The scary, red devils entered the stage. The devils picked up Jenn and proceeded to throw her, kicking and screaming, down into this fire pit. Steve's hand squeezed my leg so hard at this moment. I looked at him and mouthed, "I'm sorry." I looked at Lee, and his eyes were bugging out of his head. The preacher then entered center stage, turned up the house lights, and asked who was ready to be saved. Lee threw his hand up in the air, and I quickly pulled it down. We perspired through the parade of the newly saved. We finally escaped and sat down with the kids for a long time processing the events of the day. It was a traumatic experience for my children when it occurred. We laugh about it now.

Laughter was an important element in the family, especially when Grandma Joan or Uncle Scott was around. Uncle Scott had married a California girl and became stepdad to her three kids. Right after Lee was born, Scott brought Diana back east to Georgia to live. Through the years, we had gatherings at both our houses for friends and family for lots of the major holidays and for the typical birthday celebrations. Debbie, Mark's first wife, and their girls, Julia and Jayne, made the trip from North Carolina at least once a year. Julia and Jayne were close in age to Bonnie and Lee. Grandma loved having Bonnie, Julia, and Jayne over to her house for tea parties and slumber parties. Mark visited about once a year too, sometimes bringing Julia and Jayne, and sometimes bringing a lady friend he was seeing at the time. I welcomed him with reservation. He still went off once in a while, especially around my mom or me. When Joan on occasion complained to me about Harry or Mark, perhaps some of her poison was shifted into my being, blending with my own reserve, further hindering the health of my own connections with my father and brother.

The relationship I have with my brothers can be best described by using a pet analogy. When I am around Scott, I assume the characteristics most identified with a dog. I display trust, adoration, and eagerness to please in his presence. If I had a tail, it would wag enthusiastically when Scott entered a room. When I am around Mark, I assume the characteristics most identified with a cat. I display mistrust, nervousness, and an awareness of a need for an escape route. If I had a tail, it would twitch uneasily when Mark entered a room.

But most of the time, the family togetherness was just plain fun. Our mom had passed down the belief that laughter could push any pain out of a room, even if only momentarily. Steve especially loved Christmas time. He would be up before the kids every year. He would be all showered and dressed, fire roaring, coffee made, the video camera set up, anxiously awaiting the sleepy-headed children weaving down the hall. After the Santa-filled morning, guests would arrive. Scott and Diana and their family always entered with arms full of wine and tasty goodies. Uncle Scott bought the coolest presents like pogo sticks, Hoppity Hops, and Nerf sword fighting sets. At some moment in the afternoon, I passed out the words to the song, "Blowin' in the Wind," and made everyone sing along with Peter, Paul, and Mary's rendition. One year, Lee received a gift, a jar of slime stuff that made a farting sound when you pushed your fingers into the goop. That year during our annual singing of "Blowin' in the Wind," he produced the loud farting sound with perfect timing after each chorus of "The answer, my friend, is blowin' in the wind/The answer is blowin' in the wind." There wasn't a dry eye in the room.

In the summer, the cookouts took over. On one such occasion, while in the kitchen with my mom mixing up potato salad, Steve was quickly vacuuming the living room before the neighbors arrived. He didn't finish in time. As the little girl next door entered the house, she yelled, "I didn't know Daddies could vacuum!" Her mama gave her daddy, who wasn't much help in the house, the evil eye.

My mom whispered to me, "If a vacuum is a threat to your manhood, you're not very sure of your manhood, are you?" I giggled. Grandma Joan had a quick and highly perceptive wit.

Grandma was always there. When she traveled with us, she put on her bathing suit and swam in the ocean surf, and she rode the roller coaster, laughing all the way. She took Bonnie and her best friend Jodi to the top of the Westin Peachtree Plaza Hotel downtown every year at Christmas time. They ate lunch in the fancy revolving restaurant, and the girls exchanged their gifts over dessert. Grandma volunteered at the Fernbank Natural History Museum, and she got permission for Bonnie to join her as she fulfilled her duties. Bonnie thought she was Ms. Important in her bright blue volunteer vest. I loved the fact that Grandma could impart her wisdom to Bonnie. Joan was a great role model for Bonnie and her friends.

When Grandma came over to watch Lee because he was suspended from school in the fourth grade, she didn't scold him. She took him out for ice cream. I don't think the "positive reinforcement for antisocial behavior" hurt him that day. He probably needed it. When Lee went to Grandma's house for an afternoon, she'd take him out hiking or to the zoo. Once when he was in first grade, Lee went to Grandma's to watch a plumber repair her stopped up pipes. The plumber thought roots from the trees had found their way into the pipes causing blockage. The plumber was working at resuming the water flow and finally succeeded. Grandma and Lee were right in the middle of it all. Lee thought he had it all figured out and yelled, "Gwandma, maybe a hawd poop bwoke the woot!" Grandma laughed. I shared the story with Lee's speech teacher, and she added new words to his R sound target list.

Steve and I took advantage of the few times both kids were at Grandma's for the night. We made romantic dinners for two. We went over to a friend's house for a beer and a laugh. We put on a favorite Jackson Browne album and filled the bathtub with bubbles to prepare for a night of love. "The Pretender" played in the background. "And we'll fill in the missing colors/In each other's paint by number dreams." The candles were lit, and the tub toys were removed to make room for two. I'd lower myself into the warm water and glance over at Steve as he delivered two glasses of champagne. As I put my glass down on the edge of the tub, I silently removed the old Band-Aids that were resting there and tossed them in the trash. We giggled. Who says you can't mix child rearing and romance?

The laughter helped balance the inevitable tears that fell during the stressful times. When Lee was having a melt down or getting yelled at by an angry mom or dad, he suffered. Bonnie heard the turmoil from under her blankets and suffered too. Steve and I sometimes disagreed on how to handle Lee. Patience was being depleted and was often missing completely when we needed it for each other.

Once after an argument, I locked Steve out of our bedroom. He just picked the lock with a small screwdriver and entered with a smug expression. When he went to the garage to return the screw driver, I quickly locked him out of the house. I ran through the inside of the house locking all the outside doors, trying to beat him to each door. He ran around outside of the house trying to reach an unlocked door before I could lock it. I won, and he was locked out. Well, he picked at the garage door, trying to get in for a while. I kept calling him MacGyver. We loved that show, and Steve was very MacGyver-like. I returned to the bedroom to read my book with a smug expression on my face. He finally gave up on the garage door lock, but he flipped the circuit breakers to cut the power and put me in the dark. He went around outside to our bedroom window and scared the shit out of me. I let him in then, and we laughed so hard at our trickeries. We also couldn't remember what the argument was about that started the whole thing.

Our dedication and faithfulness to each other was real. I knew my mom was truly happy for me. Sometimes though, I felt a little guilty in my bliss when I looked at her sitting alone at our dinner table. She deserved to feel the bliss too. I questioned if her joy in witnessing two of her children retain happy marriages was really enough for her. I thought it would be nice if she could find love again, but she didn't agree. If I encouraged her to meet someone, she always said, "Not interested, Candy." She'd tell me to let it go. I wonder about that now, Mom, were you really fulfilled and happy by yourself, or did you avoid relationships out of fear, or were you just that damaged? I couldn't imagine any greater betrayal in a marriage than cheating on your spouse. I don't know how partners work through that obstacle. One night, Steve awoke to a dream in which I cheated on him. His temporary panic spurred a midnight conversation. We questioned if couples could make love again without inhibition after such circumstances. I sure was grateful for Steve's devotion.

Life was good for us. We tried not to miss the "Scenic View" signs that urged us to pull over along the journey, to stop and take in the experience more closely. Some of those moments became great life lessons. Lee was a Boy Scout for the first time in the fourth grade. Pinewood Derby was the big event in spring. Steve and Lee worked on a little car based on the guidelines found in the Boy Scout handbook. Steve gave Lee free reins when it came time for design and finishing touches. Lee painted his car black, his favorite color that year. He added orange flames near the wheels and painted a green lizard on the hood, his favorite animal that year. Steve helped with some physics knowledge of wheel alignment, weight positioning, and graphite powder lubrication. They were very pleased with the results. Friday night was the big weigh in, Saturday, the race. The father and son set off with the acclaimed Pinewood Derby car. Lee was beaming. When they returned home that night, however, something happened. Lee came in the house with his head down, looking totally deflated. "What's wrong?" I asked. Steve told me about the dads who took Pinewood Derby to a new level. There were professional paint jobs, little plastic driver men glued into a carved out seat in the body of the car, decals, spoilers, and any other cool doo-dad available, probably through some Pinewood Derby catalog. Lee thought his car looked too homemade. It was lame in comparison. Steve tried to cheer him and explained looks weren't that important. Saturday morning, we all went to the race. Lee's car kicked ass. He beat every single fancy shmancy car out there. He won the first place trophy. It was a great day.

Sometimes, the life lessons didn't end in righteous satisfaction. Once, Lee and I flew to visit my grandparents who were retired in the country about ninety miles from Buffalo. They lived in an old schoolhouse next to a farm for over thirty years. I had spent a week's vacation each summer with my mom's parents while growing up. It was such a happy memory, and I wanted to share the experience with Lee. He needed it. Other than the Pinewood Derby trophy, fourth grade was a rough year for him. This was a summer that Bonnie was going on a cruise ship vacation with her middle school Girl Scout group. Lee was ready for some good old-fashioned recharging that visiting Great Grandma and Great Grandpa could deliver. They would provide hugs, fresh, homemade meals, board games, listening ears, stories of wisdom, but never a judgment. It was paradise. We planned to repeat all of my favorite childhood activities like skipping rocks in the gentle river, walking the country road guard rail without falling off, running under the road through the drainage tunnel hollering out to hear the echo, feeding the cows, visiting the llama farm, and walking between the corn stalks in the vast fields. Great Grandpa would drive us around the countryside. Every time he passed a cemetery, he would say, "Lots of folks just dying to get in there." The dinner table would be just as I remembered, full of conversation and wit. Great Grandpa would tell Lee that he could pick his friends and he could pick his nose, but he couldn't pick his friend's nose. Great Grandma would then ask Great Grandpa if he could pick his nose, why did he pick that one. I loved watching Lee hear all the same stuff I heard when I was his age.

Well, while at their house, hiking by the neighboring farmer's garden, Lee and I came across a raccoon with one foot stuck in a trap. It was whimpering. Now, we were a suburban middle class family. We had read 250 picture books to our children containing cute, little woodland animals saving the day. We loved cute, little woodland animals. We wanted to help the poor creature. About that time, the farmer appeared. "Hey," I yelled. "You have a raccoon caught. Can you help him out?" The farmer didn't say a word. He just walked up to the big-eyed raccoon and hit him over the head as hard as he could with the shovel he was carrying. Thwack. Oh my God! Both Lee and I had big eyes now, filled to the brim with tears. We ran back to Grandma and Grandpa's house. I felt awful for not protecting Lee by foreseeing the farmer's solution which became the raccoon's demise.

It was just so matter of fact and so violent. Lee learned that farmers didn't look at cute, little woodland creatures the same way that families from the suburbs did. When I had the chance to be alone with the farmer and scold him for the brutal act my son witnessed, he just laughed at me.

Sometimes, there were some sharp curves in the road. I had always watched Bonnie's back for signs of scoliosis. Sure enough, I passed that flaw down. When it was time to go to the orthopedist, I couldn't believe it, but the doctor I saw as a teenager with my mom was still practicing and became Bonnie's doctor. I thought he was an old man twenty years before, but he looked the same at her initial visit. The daughter received the same treatment plan as the mother, that plastic, form fitting back brace. Technology hadn't advanced much this time. Her sentence was identical too, about a year full time in the brace and another year sleeping in the brace. It's hard to wear a back brace to high school, especially when all your friends are wearing the cute, tight, fashionable clothes. We provided Bonnie enough sympathy, but we avoided pity. She was fine, and we never doubted her ability to handle this setback. My parents' behavior was a good model to follow on this one. They never doubted my ability either.

Lee continued his relationships with orthopedists as well. He visited the emergency room six times before he was grown, three stitches, one broken collarbone, and four broken arms. He actually had two broken arms at the same time when he was fourteen. Lee ran a lot. He fell at school. He fell at home. By trying not to land on the arm already in a full cast, he landed on and snapped the good one. His ingenuity got a work out for the four weeks that both of his arms were in full casts. He returned to school with his two ninety degree stiff arms, one in a black cast, and one in a white cast. It's amazing what he could accomplish. It was uncomfortable for him, the things he couldn't accomplish. Dad stepped in when needed.

My mom used to say to me, "I cried when I had no shoes, until I met the man who had no feet." I certainly repeated the sentiment to my children when the situation was fitting. My mother taught me to be thankful for what I had and to notice the difficulties so many people in the world faced. I wasn't allowed to feel sorry for myself. What a great lesson to learn and then pass on to my children. It's a conscious effort to decide what lessons from your own childhood are pass-down-worthy and what parenting practices are purposefully eliminated. I don't think I thanked my parents enough for the sporadic gifts of wisdom they imparted that aided my successes. But I also didn't condemn them for their intermittent spells of faulty child rearing habits that at times impeded my successes. So Steve and I both attempted to better the parenthood design. We made sure we told our kids we loved them every day as a safeguard against our own moments of flawed management.

I often question the role of the words "I love you" and the concept of duty in this world. I think a lot about it. How important is it to hear "I love you" out loud? Does it change as we age? I wasn't raised hearing the words "I love you." I never heard them from my parents. Steve didn't hear them as a child either. I don't think it was as popular back then as it is today. I think it's important though. Kids need to hear that their parents love them. Steve and I told each other those words every day as well. I never heard my parents say "I love you" to each other. I never saw it written on a card. How unfortunate for them and for us kids.

Years ago, I had a conversation about this topic with my mom. She said she never heard those words growing up either, but she claimed she knew her parents loved her. Did she really? I don't think I could say I knew my parents loved me, especially in adolescence. My mom told me she loved me that day of our conversation, but it felt awkward. It never felt natural saying "I love you" to her or when she said it to me. So we just didn't. That's sad. She thought the words were thrown around too liberally. Isn't that better than too conservatively? She was of the opinion that the passionate Mediterranean families that shouted at each other in anger and later said, "I love you" were practicing inconsistent and strange behavior. I thought the dispassionate, stiff upper lip, WASP practice of hiding your feelings, both the good and bad feelings, was strange behavior. There's moderation somewhere in those extremes. Thankfully, my little family broke the disconnect to the words "I love you," especially after troubled times when we all really needed to hear it the most.

Yet even without the spoken words between my mom and me, duty took hold successfully throughout our adult relationship. Can duty and love be one and the same? I think of the abundant loving memories we shared. I included my mom in the life of my family. As an adult, I really did enjoy my mom's company. I took care of her without feeling it was one iota of drudgery. With her living alone for most of my adult life, that's just the way it was. Near the end, when I was doing almost everything for her, I thought about our unspoken love for each other. It made me think of the song that Tevye and Golde sang to each other in *The Fiddler on the Roof.* He was questioning her love because they never had spoken the words. She claimed her household duties were love. "If that's not love, what is?" she asked. It's confusing because duty and love look an awful lot alike. When you don't resent the duty, when it is pleasurable, is that the same as love? Does it matter? It's just something I think about sometimes, based on my experiences; other people think differently I'm sure.

Anyway, as a parent, I gained many life lessons from my children as well. I found out that it's a bad idea to just wrap the coat around your little girl and zip it without putting her arms in the sleeves when running out to the mailbox real quick on a cold winter day. Poor Bonnie tripped and fell on her face, unable to catch herself with her bound up arms. I felt so bad. Lessons in not sweating the small stuff were everywhere. Kids are messy. The white zit splats on the bathroom mirror only proved my little ones were growing up. During Lee's teen growth spurt, with my bottle of Windex and paper towel in hand, I watched those splats move ever higher up the glass. I thought about leaving them as a unique kind of growth chart.

I figured out how to be a better teacher for kids who didn't fit the mold from my son, Lee. I loved teaching the gifted, the challenged, the hyper, and the behavior problems. Kids who didn't "act right" were bombarded with negative messages from the time their feet first hit the floor in the morning until they closed their woeful eyes at night. I was going to do what I could to try and tip the balance just a bit. I remember a teacher describing with disgust the actions of a little girl in her class. "She sat there at circle time and removed her socks from her feet without removing her sandals first! She kept the sandals on, and when she had completed her task, she clutched her socks in her hands high up in the air with pride. She was supposed to listening to the story! Have you ever heard of anything so ridiculous? What a strange child." I wanted that little girl in my third grade class. I thought she sounded brilliant.

As a teacher, I saw the uneven playing field. Some students came to the classroom with the weight of their unfortunate circumstances heavy on their backs, yet some entered the classroom completely bubble wrapped. Twenty-five students each school year with disparities in appearance, wealth, intelligence, and self-control, looking up to the adult in the room, an elementary school teacher of a few years has seen it all.

On the first day of school one year when I was teaching third grade, the class was completing a word search handout containing common school terminology. The words to search for were listed at the bottom of the page, words like math, crayon, recess, and teacher. Little Michelle approached me and said, "I have found a word that often describes third grade. However, it is not listed at the bottom of the worksheet. Should I circle it anyway?"

I said, "Sure, what's the word?"

"Chaos," replied eight-year-old Michelle.

The next week we were studying birds and feathers. We were comparing and contrasting the flight feather and the down feather. The students were to observe and describe their findings. One exercise directed the students to throw the feathers up in the air and analyze the differences in the way they descended to the ground. Little Charlie ran up to me with such enthusiasm.

"Teacher, teacher, did you see? Dis one do dat, and dat one do dis."

What an uneven playing field. Vocabulary acquisition is a strong predictor of school success, and the disparity of that trait alone is overwhelming. Individualized instruction, small groups, peer teaching, teachers do it all to try and reach the whole class, from the Michelles to the Charlies. One simple step to improve school performance parents should practice is to read to their children every chance they get. I'd like to start an R2K movement. Read 2000 books to your children by kindergarten. Reading provides vocabulary building, problem solving, science and social studies content, empathy development, and most importantly, emotional bonding between parent and child. It quickly became clear to me that a child's ability to be successful in school wasn't just about good teaching strategies and school budgets. And parents who didn't read to their children were only the tip of the iceberg. Sadly, it's difficult for them to learn anything when children are neglected, abused, tired, hungry, scared, or angry.

Mario was a new student in my fourth grade class. He had a long discipline record. We used to walk around the track and talk during recess. I liked Mario. I met Mario's mother for a parent teacher conference to discuss his progress. She didn't ask me what she could do *for* Mario; she asked me what she could do *with* Mario. She didn't want him anymore. She was scared and couldn't handle him any longer. I referred Mario to our counselor who supplied the mother with some resources. Mario's mother said she had heard it all before. She really just wanted to be rid of him. I wondered how something that started out so wonderful could end up so horrible. Mario moved into a group home. I wound up back in college. After teaching for ten years, my educational interests were leaning more toward the affective growth of my students rather than the cognitive growth. I returned to Georgia State University to obtain a Master's degree to become a school counselor.

I always talked to my mom about school, the students, the trends, my joys and frustrations. She loved hearing about my career. She helped me come up with some great lesson plans sometimes. She would have made a wonderful elementary school teacher. She was the best Sunday School teacher at the Congregational church when we lived in Vermont. Her artistic creativity was everywhere. For her class, she ordered chicken eggs and an incubator every Easter, so they could experience the hatching of baby chicks. I loved visiting her room, listening to the chirping sounds, and holding the fluffy chicks. It's funny; she never suggested I become a teacher when I was growing up. But the concrete belief in the importance of respecting children was handed down to me by my mom, and that made me a better teacher and counselor.

One of my first small group counseling sessions was targeting kindergarten boys with poor listening skills. We were sitting around the table introducing ourselves. I asked them to go around the circle and tell everyone their name. The first little boy said, "Juan." I looked at the second little boy, Jeffrey. He just looked at me, very unsure of what he was supposed to do. I guess he didn't listen. After a few seconds, he said, "Two?"

Little kids will tell their counselor lots. They reveal what they heard Mommy and Daddy screaming about the night before. They draw pictures of the fear they feel when Daddy hits Mommy. They cry in your office when their parents are getting divorced. They tell you how the bruises really got on their leg and arm. I thought about the trials of my own youth and how difficult some of my paths to healing proved to be. How would these children fare, with obstacles that were far more painful and damaging than anything I ever experienced? I worried for their future. They needed more safety nets along their journey. We have to do more as a society to reduce the abuses of children. The job of elementary school counselor is not for the fainthearted, and I persevered at it for four years.

When the Governor of Georgia decided to address the high school dropout rate by adding an extra counselor to each high school, I accepted a new job. This counseling position's charge was to try and help the at-risk kids, to provide extra encouragement, so they would ultimately reach graduation. High school would be a big change for me, but I had some familiarity with my own kids' experiences in high school, and I liked teenagers. I felt I could interject some acceptance and direction in this high expectation, big consequence world kids were now facing. It was also becoming harder to get up off the floor ten times a day. Elementary school teachers and counselors spend a lot of time sitting "crisscross applesauce" on the floor.

I discovered that high school kids were very similar to elementary kids, just bigger and less enthusiastic about learning, unfortunately. The problems remained the same, but anger instead of fear showed up as their favorite emotion. Working only with the students at risk for drop out simply reinforced the notion of our social ills as barriers to learning. Until we do better with neglect, abuse, poverty, violence, teen pregnancy, and drugs, we won't have a meaningful graduation rate. For me, back to basics, or the new bandwagon, rigor, isn't the only answer. The higher expectations and zero tolerances have also come at a time when society is offering an increasing number of opportunities for bad choices. Many students have single parents and less supervision, many must work to provide for their families, many are bombarded with sexual and violent images in media, and many have seen drug abuse and gun shots first hand. Did I say we need to take better care of our children?

Big kids tell their counselor lots too. The stories broke my heart. Jade was a fifteen year old with two kids of her own trying to continue her education. Maria was a sixteen year old who was raped, but felt maybe it was her fault because she sneaked out that night. Felina was a seventeen year old whose parents drank, fought, moved away, and left her alone to fend for herself. Nan was a fifteen year old with braces on her teeth and a cocaine habit. Erika was an undocumented student whose mother was facing a court date. Erika was afraid her mother might be deported, and she was worried about having to take care of her younger siblings and remain in school. Mike, the baseball player, was having a problem with skittles, the cold medicine pill that got him high when he swallowed twelve at a time. Brandy, the high achieving orchestra student, cut herself to see her pain. Shayla was a fourteen year old who went home and babysat three little brothers alone every day until her mom came home from work at ten o'clock expecting a spotless house and perfect grades. Jake was the boy who had trouble dealing with the fact that his Grandmother must raise him because both of his parents were on drugs. Shane had a gun under his bed and was afraid of the day he might use it. And then, there was Lance, who wore the home detention monitor ankle bracelet on his leg while attending high school classes. For the "greatest" country in the world, there sure are a lot of young people in pain.

I didn't get to talk much to my mom about this new career path. We were well into the Alzheimer's dilemma when I took the job of high school counselor. I so much missed that opportunity to use her as a sounding board. Joan was always so wise and continuously complimentary of my endeavors.

Chapter 12   The Drugs

The phone rang at six thirty in the morning on the fifth of February. It was Country Gardens. "Candy, you have to come get your mom. She is scaring the residents, and we can't stop her. She's talking crazy. She's out of control."

I called in to work to let them know I wouldn't be there that day. I drove over to Country Gardens and arrived about seven fifteen. I walked down the corridor to reach Joan's room. She was in her pajamas, her hair sticking up all over the place, and she was in a crazed state of panic. "Candy, oh my God! The heater is putting out this deadly gas! All of the people who live here have been taken out on stretchers! They are all in the hospital! The gas is killing them! Oh my God! They all went to the hospital in ambulances. The gas is killing me. It's coming from my heater over there." The nurse's aide on duty just looked at me. Joan had been up all night in this state of panic.

I asked the aide what I should do. She said I could call her doctor or take her to the hospital. I got Joan dressed and took her home with me. I called her neurologist, but the hour was before the office opened, so I left a message. Steve called me to check in, and I told him I'd let him know soon what we were going to do. Joan sat on my couch and stared at me. She stood up and walked in a circle. She sat back down. Her eyes were not those of the woman I used to call Mom. If I tried to engage in conversation, she just looked at me with a wide-eyed expression of confusion and distress. She kept getting up and walking around my house looking for mirrors. She stopped at each mirror to have a conversation with the woman in the reflection. She usually used a whisper voice. "She likes me. No, she hates me. Why does she hate her mother? I don't know." The mirror talking was really creepy.

I called the doctor again. They were now open, and the receptionist answered. But when I was forwarded to the nurse's desk, I reached another answering machine and was asked to leave another message. Joan continued to walk around my house stopping at every mirror to whisper some sort of madness to her reflection. I was scared. She stared at her own face in the mirror and used that chilling whisper voice. "And he said he would be right back. He did. He did. Harry said he'd be right back. That's what he told me." Then, she would break into a yell. "HE NEVER CAME BACK! HARRY NEVER CAME BACK!" She was the craziest I've ever seen anyone before, Hollywood movie crazy. I had never before felt fear in the presence of my own mother until that day. I didn't know this person. Her eyes were possessed. I started thinking about exorcisms. I started thinking about strait jackets, frontal lobotomies, and other mental hospital stuff. The nurse from the doctor's office finally returned my call around ten o'clock. I told her everything that was happening. She said she would talk to the doctor and get back to me. I asked her to please hurry, to please call right back. We hung up.

Joan decided to start arguing with me about going to church. Jesus seems to be an important item on the menu of despair, especially for those facing life sentences in prison, those with terminal illnesses, or those just nearing death. Maybe they're looking for Him, or maybe He's looking for them. So she yelled at me to go to church. My mother taught me to be open-minded and accepting of all lifestyles, ideologies, beliefs, and faiths, including the faithless. Usually, her receptive and curious nature bore validity to a number of alternative thoughts, both individual and cultural thoughts. Of course, like most of us, at certain times on certain issues, her mind was very opinionated. It's strange how it works that way. Nevertheless, we had engaged in many conversations about our acceptance of and the authenticity of all world religions. We had talked about the purpose, the roots, and the need of religion throughout the history of civilization, and how spirituality continued to evolve. We acknowledged the inconsistency in Bible interpretation. The Catholics had a gambling and beer party, casino night, as a church fundraiser. The Baptists disallowed drinking, gambling, or dancing. They both read the same book. We used to be on the same page. Now here she was, screaming at me over and over because I didn't go to church. My mom, who had lost her sanity, wanted me to find religion.

I finally told her I did go to church, which wasn't really a lie, and it calmed her somewhat. I told her I went to the Chattahoochee River Church. Steve and I take our kayaks or our canoe out on the river many Sunday mornings. We paddle up stream for exercise and then float downstream for relaxation. We marvel at the calm beauty of the river in the morning. We witness and express wonder at the kingfishers, the herons, the ducks, the woodpeckers, the songbirds, the muskrats, the squirrels, and the turtles basking in the sun. We gaze in awe at the mist suspended above the water and the blue sky over our heads. We become re-energized with the beauty of the earth, whether a God, a Big Bang, or Mother Nature brought it to us. We enjoy life together. That's church for us, and those few hours each week help us cope. I recognize how often nature has been my calm and my strength. My news seemed to slow down her rants but not completely satisfy her. She went to the bathroom to whisper about me to her reflection in the mirror. "She is going to get fired. Her principal told me that. He said Candy couldn't work there anymore. She doesn't go to church."

By ten thirty the phone hadn't rung, and I was beginning to shake. I called my brother Scott at work to tell him what was going on. I started to cry. I told him I hoped to hear back from the doctor soon, and Scott asked me to keep him posted. I called Steve at work. I cried to him my tears of fear, fatigue, and complete helplessness. He responded with, "I'll be right there." For over ten years, Steve had been working in management for an automotive service warranty company that was owned by a man who believed in a balance of hard work and family time. Steve's passion for bending over car engines waned at forty, and he was now thriving in his new vocation as a white collar worker. His fingernails were finally clean. He arrived home quickly, and his presence got me through. Why did I think I could get through this alone? I had to admit how scary the situation was. I really couldn't do it by myself. I felt so much better when Steve pulled up, unbelievable relief. Joan continued to angrily walk around the house speaking to her reflection in the mirrors using those vile whispering and yelling voices. Together, Steve and I waited for the phone to ring, and we watched the performance, a one-woman show.

At eleven thirty, the doctor's office called back. The neurologist's nurse asked me if she was taking her Aricept and that maybe she needed some more. WHAT? That was the information I had been waiting over three hours to hear, more Aricept? Had she been listening at all to what I described to her? I think I yelled at the nurse. I think I told her how ridiculous that suggestion was. Any stages of anger I may have experienced through this whole ordeal of loss and grief usually involved the medical field.

I called Country Gardens back. I asked the aide who answered the phone what children did for their parents who were going through this experience. She must have seen this type of thing before. She gave me the name of a geriatric mental health hospital some of the residents had worked with. I was familiar with the hospital because it was located in the same town we lived in for eighteen years, where we raised our family. I called the hospital. I talked to a nice receptionist who took my information and said someone would get back to me soon. Steve and I ate lunch with the deranged woman named Joan.

At one o'clock a nurse called from the geriatric mental health hospital. My description of Joan matched their hospital's function. She had sensed the urgency in my voice and tried to reassure me all would be fine. She said she needed a doctor's approval to admit Joan. I gave her Joan's doctor's number. We waited some more for her to call us back. Joan started to calm down and fell asleep for a little bit. At three o'clock the nurse called again with an approval, but by this time it was too late to get Joan in to the mental health hospital that same day. We had an appointment for nine thirty the next morning. This nice woman gave me all the instructions and procedures for committing your mother to a mental hospital. After we hung up, Steve and I were trying to think about how we could make it through the night with Joan. Did we need her to stay with us for the night? How could I take her back to Country Gardens?

At three thirty the phone rang again. It was the neurologist's office. They came through with a prescription for an antipsychotic drug to help Joan make it through the night. Maybe that nice lady at the mental health hospital told Joan's doctor to call me back with something more helpful than more Aricept. Steve went to the drugstore to get the pill that would help us make it through the night. I called Scott to fill him in on one of the worst days of my life.

We decided to take Joan back to Country Gardens for dinner, a pill, and bed. She had to be exhausted. Scott planned on meeting us there. Her craziness had subsided by the time he arrived. She was actually playful with Scott. I don't think he understood the dose of hell I had experienced that day. He had never seen her in the mirror lady role. We ate dinner with her and told her she needed to bathe before bed because she had an appointment with Dr. Pat the next morning. She asked, "Who?"

"Dr. Pat," I repeated.

"Who?" she asked again.

"Dr. Pat," I said.

"Spell it," she said.

"P – A – T."

"T – P – A?"

"No, P – A – T."

"T – A – P?"

"No, Dr. Pat."

She picked up a pen and wrote down Dr. Pate. We all left her with the pill in the hands of the night nurse. Scott shook his head on the way down the hall.

The next morning arrived too quickly. I again called in to work, explained the situation, and drove to Country Gardens. While Joan finished her breakfast in the dining hall, I packed her overnight bag. I had all her important insurance and identification papers in a folder already. I was following the directions the geriatric mental health hospital receptionist had given me the day before. I hid the bag behind me as I helped Joan to the car. Explaining that she would be staying at the hospital for a while would be fruitless. She would forget that fact before we left the parking lot. Her reaction could also be unpredictable, from an approving nod to an unhinged rant. I didn't want to take any chances.

At first, Joan was in good spirits that day. We arrived at the hospital on time. We filled out papers, answered questions, and produced the important documents. A psychologist took her to another room for a little while to complete a short assessment. They took her blood pressure and tried to weigh her. She decided that she didn't want to get on the scale. She was just like our dog when we try to get him in the bathtub, total resistance. They did the best they could. Next, a nurse took her to another room for a picture. When Joan returned from the photo shoot, she approached me with her whisper voice. "They won't let me have any of the pictures. When Candy asked for a picture of me, they said no, no, no, you can't have a picture of your mother. Candy can't have any pictures of her mother." I just looked at her and said nothing.

They emptied the contents of her overnight bag into a brown paper bag and wrote her name on the outside with a black, permanent marker. That just seemed so impersonal. Her name was already on all of her clothes, a directive in place from Country Gardens living. They informed me of the visiting hours, twelve to two and six to eight, and discouraged me from visiting too soon. They put her in a wheel chair and took her away. I didn't get to go with my mom to see where they were taking her. I didn't get to explain anything to her. I felt so terribly sneaky and dishonest. She was like a small child with no one to protect her. I had been protecting her for quite some time. I had accompanied her to all of her medical appointments for years and was always allowed to stay with her through the visits. It was an awful feeling leaving her alone. I walked to the parking lot with her empty overnight bag in my hand and tears in my eyes.

Steve and Bonnie were in the parking lot waiting for me. I had checked in with Steve periodically during the morning. He called Bonnie, and they both took the afternoon off from work. We all went to a late lunch, and they tried to cheer me. We returned to the hospital right before the afternoon visiting hours were over, but the receptionist told us to leave, to give it some time. She used the reasoning that it would be too hard on Joan and on us. She was very persuasive, and we all went home. I was exhausted.

Scott went against the hospital's suggestion that we wait a while before visiting, and he visited Joan that same night whereupon he received his dose of hell. They put Mom in a high security wing. They called it the high flight risk wing. The big double doors were locked. There were crazy people in the halls yelling, crying, laughing, and just making random noises. Every human emotion was displayed in that small wing of a hospital, absent of visible context. Men and women were together banging on doors, pacing, crouching in corners, and even running up and down the hall. They were in various stages of dress, some in hospital gowns, some in underwear, some in street clothes, unzipped or unbuttoned, one sock on, and one sock off. Scott was heartbroken. Mom was terrified in there. There were doctors and nurses everywhere with clipboards and pens in hand. Apparently, this was an "observation" period. Mom had a room with no door as did everyone else locked up on this hall, and no one knew which room was theirs. She was sitting on a rubber-lined bed with Scott when a crazy man walked in mumbling. Mom was jumpy and scared. She begged Scott to get her out of there. She was crying to him, "How can you leave me in a place like this? What are you doing to me? I want to leave this place right now. I want to go home." She clung to him when visiting hours were over. Scott called me on his way home to fill me in on one of the worst days of his life. In this case, her sanity was harder to bear than her insanity.

We talked a lot about this decision. It was clearly dreadful. Scott said that if you weren't crazy when you entered that place, it would make you crazy in a moment's time. We were told this was the process. What could we have done differently? Where else do you get help for mentally failing, old folks? There was no way we could take her on ourselves. We had to go to work every day. Scott commented that rich people didn't go through this type of treatment. We started thinking about what people did in the old days with the mad. Put Grandma in the birthing/dying room with a bottle of whiskey, over a cliff, insane asylums, or rubber rooms? Mom used to kid about growing old back when she was vibrant. She said when it was her time to go, when she lost her ability to be independent, she would like to go over the railing of a cruise ship into the sea with a gin and tonic in her hand. Scott and I often joked about booking a cruise the last year or so throughout this whole ordeal.

We had no choice really but to trust the system. I visited the next evening after work, very unprepared to meet my new mom. Joan didn't plead with me. Her will was gone, replaced by drugs. She was in a stupor. She walked the halls like the people that had been there for more than a few days in a glazed-eyed, over-medicated state. She had dried food on her chin. She had her slippers on the wrong feet. Her hair was flattened on one side. She didn't speak at all. It was almost too much to bear. Tragic. The doctors and nurses said this was the "medicine adjustment" period. They had to see what kinds of drugs worked, what dose was best. I could attest that they still had work to do with Joan. I hugged her unresponsive, stiff body and left, fighting back the tears until I reached the car. The series of goodbyes continued, and the goodbye that day was by far the worst to date. Joan was gone.

Scott complained to the staff about the placement of Joan in the most restrictive wing. After a couple of days, they moved her into the moderate flight risk wing forty feet to the left. It was so sad to walk by that first hall she occupied for a short time. There was always a face in the window of the door, peering out with panicked eyes. It took fifteen days for the hospital to concoct what they felt was the best psychotropic cocktail for Joan's condition. During that time, Scott and I visited her every day, alternating evenings. It was a little better in her new wing. It was a calmer hall but still depressing. I began to recognize many of the familiar faces. Scott and I would discuss the patients, giving them names, crying lady, mad lady, and racist man. Maybe some dominant emotion or feeling found in a sane person would take over completely when they became insane, the regulation switch broken. The mad lady was always grumbling. The sad lady was always weeping. The racist man was painfully insulting to the nurse trying to feed him. I apologized to her for his behavior. I don't know how she maintained professionalism. Joan became a mute, but Mom talked all the time in her previous life. It's hard to make sense of the senseless.

The doctor couldn't come up with any reason for Joan's refusal to talk. When he reduced the amount of the medications, allowing for more reality to seep through, she would become combative, his exact word. The purpose of the drugs was to keep her anxiety and hallucinations under control, but at the same time, her confusion from Alzheimer's never faltered. It seemed like no one was exactly sure what was going on with Joan's mental health. If the doctors did know anything, they seldom shared with the patient's family. Communication with the family was inadequate. Questions for the doctors were met with uncertainty. Her brain was just messed up and treated with experimental drug concoctions.

One day when I arrived, she was in someone else's room, not unusual. She had on someone else's clothes, however, which was a new trick. She sported a bold flowered shirt, black slacks, and a lacy, 38 double D,

Cross Your Heart Bra. Joan weighed about eighty-five pounds at this point, and none of the weight was in her chest. I laughed and asked her where she got the clothes. She just stared at me expressionless. I found the owner of the pretty outfit and got Mom back in her own attire.

The visits during her time in this hospital were short. We walked down the hall, looked out the window, and sat on a couch. As the medication regulated through her system, she sometimes could muster up a sentence or two. I told her about my life and the kids' lives anyway. Maybe on some level she understood and enjoyed these conversations. One story I told her every time I visited was about the time that she had been in this place before. The building used to be a small, general hospital where both of my children happened to be born. After a newer and bigger hospital was built nearby, the facility became home to a number of different medical services, currently this geriatric mental health hospital. Joan just stared at me when I said, "Mom, this is the same wing and everything. This is where you watched your granddaughter come into the world. Remember being in the room with us, Mom? You just stood in the background and watched the whole episode with amazement, Steve and Candy working so hard together to reach the ultimate goal of parenthood. It was an amazing experience for you, and here you are in the same place now."

I'm not certain every woman would be comfortable with her own mother being present during her childbirth experience. But something occurred earlier in my life to want me to include my mom in this wondrous event. When I was twenty, my friend Kim found herself with child and without man. She chose to have and keep her baby. She asked me to be her labor coach, and I said,

"Sure!" I was working nights at the time, so we could attend all her Lamaze classes together. I found it all very cool. On the day of her delivery, I was fully enthralled with Kim's courageous efforts and mesmerized by my encounter with birth. I don't think there was anything I had witnessed in my life to that point that was as fascinating as watching Kim's child enter the world. When my responsibility was through for the night, I stopped by Manuel's Tavern, our local bar, to tell Lea Anne and everyone who knew Kim all the details of the happy event. I woke up my mom when I got home to chatter endlessly about all the particulars, and I called Steve up in Canada very late to share the news too. I was high for days.

When it was my turn at pregnancy, I knew my mom had never experienced childbirth as a spectator, so I wanted her to see the joy from that perspective. I'm not sure she found the experience as exhilarating as I did, probably because it's hard to watch your own daughter struggle with so much pain. But I'm glad I asked my mom to be present, and I'm glad she said, "Sure!"

Thankfully, Steve went to the hospital to see Mom with me on weekends to make it less dreadful. Bonnie visited a couple of times too, driving up from school. She was excited to share her recent news of an engagement. She showed Grandma her ring, and Grandma smiled. We talked to Joan a lot about getting better, so she could dance and carry on at Bonnie's wedding planned for October. Grandma smiled again and whispered, "I want to go." I knew she wanted to be there more than anything. I also knew how much Bonnie wanted her there. Shit, it was sad. I think it's called the bargaining stage when we silently wish for something we know won't really happen. We were all sister-less, my mom, me, and my daughter. We missed out on that special bond sisters sometimes share. We created a type of multi-generational sisterhood to fill our void, and it worked for us. Now, we were losing a link.

So after these two weeks were up, the doctor felt he had reached the best he could do with Joan's mental health, and she returned to Country Gardens. Things were different then. She didn't talk much or interact with any of her neighbors. She didn't participate in the life at Country Gardens. She stared blankly at nothing, and her chin became an out of control pendulum, swinging back and forth. A habit, or side effect, that came with the new meds was an oscillating chin. We would put our hand on her chin to stop the movement, and as soon as we released the grip, it would start up again.

Scott and I continued our visits, thankful to return to the more pleasant and comfortable surroundings of her apartment rather than the sterile and cold surroundings we left behind at the hospital. I didn't miss the forty mile round trip to the hospital either. But I met people there who were traveling one hundred miles to visit mothers and fathers in that hospital. And I met only children with no siblings to help them deal with the sickness of their parent. I was thankful for my family and for Country Gardens. I was also reminded of how often my mom pointed out to me the difficulties of others, wanting me to be aware of their situations. How could I complain when so many people endured far greater challenges? She encouraged me to look at the bright side if I was facing a difficulty. Those beliefs were a powerful coping mechanism. Optimism is a great gift.

In one way, medicated Joan was easier to handle for the workers at Country Gardens. She was so quiet now. She didn't complain about anything, nor did she ask for anything. But like before, she continued on with the downward momentum toward failing health. We watched her give up on life. She hardly ate anything at all, and she was losing precious weight. She stayed in her room and paced back and forth. She quit taking care of herself. I now added bathing her to my routine. She resisted, and I insisted. This was only one of many situations of blatant role reversal I found myself engaged in with my mom during her life with advanced Alzheimer's or whatever form of mental illness she possessed.

One day, I walked with her out to the communal room adjoining the dining room. A resident named Brenda asked Joan a question. Joan just stared ahead and didn't answer her. Brenda snapped, "What's the matter with you? Don't you understand English?" I walked Joan back to her room. She didn't seem to be fazed by Brenda's rudeness, but it broke my heart. I wanted to deck Brenda a big one. Just like an innocent child in need of protection and care, that was our Joan.

Joan picked up some new behaviors in her new stupor state. She started blowing her nose in her hands without the benefit of tissues. She didn't answer her door when someone knocked. The connection between knocking and entering had vanished. She sometimes would take her clothes off at inopportune moments and locations. She'd just start stripping down. You could tell when her medication was wearing off because she would reenter the lunacy world and tell her tales. She told Scott that I was stealing her money. She told him I said she was going to die on her eightieth birthday.

We had a party for her at my house on her eightieth birthday on the seventh of April. It was a beautiful spring day, azaleas in full bloom, dogwoods out. Members of the family came for a cookout, and Joan walked around in her zombie-like state. I made her favorite chocolate and cherry cake. When we sang "Happy Birthday" to her and presented her with the candles for blowing out, she smiled and said, "I like cherries." We all cheered and blew her candles out for her. She forgot how to do that part.

In May, we had a party for Bonnie's graduation from Georgia College and State University. Joe, Lee, Scott and Diana, Lea Anne and her husband were all there. Dad and Doris came too. Joan was present in body only. She kept staring at Harry. She kept taking his drink out of his hand and taking a sip. She stood really close to him and just stared blankly at his face. I bet she freaked him out completely. He looked very uncomfortable and nervous. Dad had not seen much of the mother of his children since they divorced so long ago. Shit, he hadn't seen his children or grandchildren but twice a year either. He stayed away. Was it guilt or disinterest? I'm not sure. He simply made a new life. I can't say I made an effort to include him in much though. My loyalties were with my mom. His presence made her uncomfortable, so we complied. I brought the kids to his house on the lake once each summer, and we planned a Christmas gathering together the week before the holiday each year. That was pretty much the extent of it. He told me one time that he was pleased I took such good care of my mom and that he was glad she was such a big part of my family life. I couldn't tell if his relief was driven by selfishness because it let him was off the hook or selflessness because he really cared, but I think it might have been selflessness. I think I saw a little remorse in his expression that day. Then again, it may have been my wishful thinking or a fantasy. Anyway, I had provided him with Mom's health updates during our infrequent phone conversations over the past few years, describing her recent mental decline.

So we all had as nice a time as we could during this celebration day. We talked a lot about the upcoming wedding. We all watched the home video of Bonnie receiving her diploma. She looked right into the camera immediately after shaking hands with the university president and smiled. Joe asked her how she knew where her dad would be standing with the camera. She explained that all her life her Dad was always at the best vantage point at every game, milestone, award night, recital, performance, and celebration to capture the significant event. I often complained about being a video widow. I sat through many such events with my mom and without Steve. I used to tease him that he was missing out on the enjoyment of the moment as he planned and fulfilled his video capture. I thought he was crazy to place preference on watching these events later on the television set in his living room. But I must confess that reliving these childhood memories through family videos is beyond awesome. I treasure the home movies with all my heart and can watch them over and over. Steve was right again.

After returning Joan to Country Gardens that night, we sat around a little longer and talked about her decline in health. We were used to the mental decline, but she was really losing her physical strength now too. Joan was becoming weaker day by day and consequently was becoming unsteady on her feet. She fell down a couple of times, unbelievably not injuring herself. Her behavior and physical condition scared me. She had held on for three months at Country Gardens in her new dulled state before further interventions were once again necessary.

Very early in the morning on May 26, Country Gardens called. Joan couldn't stand up and walk without support, but she refused to sit still. They couldn't have someone right next to her twenty-four hours a day, and they were worried about her falling and breaking a bone. She needed more than they could provide. They wanted me to come get her. This was the day of the high school graduation ceremony that I was to be a part of at twelve o'clock noon. I called Scott to arrange the details of time management, so I could attend to Joan and attend my school's graduation ceremony. I was told to take Joan to the emergency room first, and from there she could return to the same geriatric mental health hospital she had been to before. So while I got ready in my dress up clothes, Steve ironed my graduation gown. I picked Joan up an hour after the Country Gardens phone call for a trip to the emergency room. Scott was going to meet us there at eleven o'clock, so I could leave for a while, only to return to her again in the late afternoon. Hopefully by then, she would be settled at her old, familiar, crazy house stomping grounds once more. I didn't really know what they could do to resolve this situation. In this helpless state, you just sort of do what you are told by those in charge.

Joan and I sat in the emergency waiting room for a while. I mostly kept my hands over her lap to prevent her from getting up and falling down. Her name was called, and all the usual emergency room tests began. She was a good patient. When it became time for the urine sample, she needed assistance. I got to hold the cup while Joan peed.

Scott relieved me in the late morning, and I attended the high school graduation ceremony. As soon as it was over, I called Scott. They were settling in at the mental health hospital. I drove straight there to see them both. Most of the staff remembered Joan, and we were right back in the routine of life in the old folks' mental hospital. For whatever ailed you, they had the antidote. She was treated for dehydration. They ordered a new drug to increase her appetite. She began eating pureed food which helped her get more calories down. They were set on making her stronger. They adjusted her meds. These interventions helped a bit, but a new side effect or habit was troublesome. Mom started putting her head down at a ninety degree angle. She walked around with her head completely folded over, eyes aimed on the floor. The doctor ordered an X-ray to see if something in her neck was broken, but results showed nothing wrong. If they put a neck brace on her, she tore it off. This was just the way it was. A drooping head replaced the oscillating chin.

I was out of school and finished with work for the year, free. Summers off were a delicious perk for me. Attending to Joan's needs became easier in some ways. Having more time to process what was going on in our lives was also a curse. You know how it feels when you stay reclined in the bathtub after a warm soak and let the water drain out of the tub? You go through the funky sensation of warm buoyancy and almost weightlessness gradually changing to a cold, awkward heaviness as gravity wins and the last drop of water exits down the drain. There is an element of pleasure to the experience. But in the end, you just feel way heavy and way cold when the water is gone. It was like that. I felt capable and re-energized with the additional time I could spend with Joan at first, and then the heaviness and chill consumed me.

I had an emotional, sobbing, mini-breakdown of my own that summer. It was brief, but real, probably my biggest experience with the depression stage of grief and loss. Watching your mom in that helpless state, the mom who used to be so strong and independent, just plain sucked. She was so pitiful. Perhaps my tears freed some weight; my wails released some cold. In any case, I had little time for additional breakdowns. I just kept trying to model the strength she demonstrated throughout her life. I guess she prepared me for this, and clearly, she was worthy of my care. Joan was a beautiful and kind soul nearing the end of her life. She never deserved the pain she was dealt. If I could bring to her any amount of sunshine, it was my pleasure.

So this trip to the hospital again took the doctors two weeks for stabilization. For six of those days I left for a previously planned vacation to Hawaii with Steve and the kids. Harry gave his children a week of his time share every now and then. We took it. I wasn't completely comfortable leaving, but I was luckily able to escape and genuinely had a blast with my family. Mark came for a visit that week to see Mom and help Scott. Scott talked to Mark periodically keeping him up to date on our lives. One of us was with her for a time each day of her stay.

The day she was to be released again, I went to get her. I walked down the hall, my head high with purpose in my step, ready to take her home to Country Gardens.

After Joan removed the men's slippers she was wearing, and we returned them to the nurse on duty so she could find the rightful owner, we put on her real shoes and went out to the parking lot. Joan returned to Country Gardens in June with a few more medications on her long list and a little more strength in her tiny body.

We walked up to the front porch where all the residents were sitting in a circle participating in an activity suited for the very young or the very old. They all cheered and yelled hello to Joan. The told her they missed her. It was so sweet, and Joan smiled for the first time in a long time. I loved that moment. People need people. Joan's big smile proved she was not completely gone. She settled back in her room.

With her back at her comfortable apartment and my summer break from work, I changed my visiting schedule. I went to see her in late morning and ate lunch with her every day. She wasn't eating much. I tried to assist by requesting the food to be delivered to her room instead of eating in the dining room, so I could help her and encourage her to eat more. The role reversals were becoming more marked. I was feeding her and even tried the "Open up, here comes the airplane" trick moms used on their children. I had a napkin in one hand to wipe her chin and a tissue in the other hand to wipe her ever-dripping nose. I still got her in the shower, every day now, because she was beginning to have accidents. We had to go out and buy adult diapers and baby wipes.

Unfortunately, only a week passed, and she was right back to falling down, returning to her weakened state before the hospital pep revival. The Country Gardens staff and I scrutinized Joan's health and behavior. The situation hadn't really improved much. They had to call the paramedics at one point after a nasty fall. She had a bump on her head. When I arrived, the emergency technician was trying to get answers from her. She was mute that day. It was becoming obvious that the assisted living facility was not a match for her needs any longer.

I called Dr. Pat who had been treating her at the mental health hospital. He approached me with little hope. He explained that Hospice was probably the next step. He did say, however, that there was one more treatment he could try. ECT, or electroconvulsive therapy, sometimes had positive results for elderly patients who suffered mental disorders stemming from depression. He asked if Joan was ever depressed. I didn't think so. She never displayed any typical symptoms of that disease. She was such an energetic and positive person, successful with work, friends, and family. But I had wondered sometimes if Mom got Alzheimer's because of the bitterness she harbored for years toward Harry. Her anger and resentment were well hidden inside, rarely shown to the outside world. But sometimes, I wondered if those feelings could have been the nourishment for the craziness that incubated and developed in her brain. Stress isn't good for emotional health. Like I said, you are always looking for the why, and maybe there just is no why. I told the doctor I would discuss this option, electric shock, with my brother, Scott.

Scott and I both agreed to try this one last attempt. How do you accept the death sentence when the doctor says there is one more option that might possibly bring your mom's brain back to some form of normalcy? We made arrangements with the doctor to return Joan to his hospital one more time. And Scott also agreed that Mom didn't suffer from depression.

A bad day was in store. It started with the car ride to the hospital. Joan kept blowing her nose in her hands. I was trying to drive and scold her and throw tissue at her most of the way. She also was reaching for the car door handle to open the door while we were en route. Even when the door was locked, it still could be opened from the inside. I continually had to lean over her and grab her hand to keep her from opening the door and falling out while I was driving. It's amazing we didn't wreck. It took mindfulness to foresee the complications that would arise while attending to her needs. I should have learned from previous experiences to take someone with me when dealing with Joan. But it was too late that day.

When we arrived, I found out that the doctor didn't communicate to the hospital's admissions department the contents of our recent conversation. Admissions had no idea we were coming, and they proceeded to tell me that there was no room for Joan. My panic mode exploded. I was trying to keep my mom from walking around to avoid a fall. I was still throwing tissues at her as she continued to blow her nose in her hands. I was arguing with the front desk administrator, pleading my case. I was trying to get this woman to call the doctor as he had sent me there. She said, "I'm sorry about that. Doctors often forget to check with admissions. We have no beds."

I sat us down in the waiting room and cried. I was actually wailing. It was too much to handle alone. Why didn't I get someone to come with me? People were staring at us. I had nowhere to go. Country Gardens wouldn't keep her, and I couldn't take her, and now, the mental hospital refused her. It was a mess. Joan was oblivious to the situation. She just looked at me expressionless as I sobbed. It's unnatural to be so upset with your mom sitting right next to you, emotionless, not even noticing your tears or not even trying to display any soothing actions. Mothers soothe their children instinctively. I just cried harder with this additional realization. Finally, the director walked into the lobby. She recognized us from our previous visits. I don't know if it was a coincidence or if security called her, but she arranged to get my mom in right away. I thanked her in between those crying breaths we all experience after wailing, three rapid inhales and one long exhale.

It was June 18. Joan had to go through a series of tests to see if she was a candidate for ECT. Her heart had to be strong enough. She had just developed a nasty cough that needed to be cleared up first. She was receiving interventions to re-hydrate her body and to put weight on her bones once again. When the preliminary procedures were completed, and she proved to be strong enough, they could begin treatment. All this took time. Joan had absolutely no understanding of what was about to happen. It was scary, and it didn't feel right a lot of the time. Second-guessing had become a past time of mine. It's a heavy load we shared, Scott and I, making decisions for Joan's health. Would she have wanted to go through with this? Each day that passed amplified my feelings of doubt.

The shock treatments had to be spaced apart with two per week. They wanted to do a series of five to eight before judging the effectiveness. Joan was in the hospital for four weeks this time. Scott and I continued to take turns checking on her almost every day throughout this time. I tried to care for my own mental health more efficiently. Steve and I talked a lot, went out on dates to a dinner or a movie, escaped with cocktails on the lower deck, threw ourselves into home improvement projects to prepare for Bonnie's wedding, and he held me closer at night.

It was the summer of alternating and contrasting activities. The planning of Bonnie and Joe's wedding was occurring simultaneously with Joan's health care issues. Keeping busy is in itself a way to cope. One day was spent walking Joan up and down the hospital halls, the next day, making wedding invitations with Bonnie at the dining room table. One day was spent feeding Joan her pureed food, the next day, painting the basement to prepare for a wedding celebration. One day was spent talking to doctors about medication, the next day, talking to caterers about appetizers. On good days, the fun wedding plans became a positive diversion to the sadness of my mom's circumstances. On bad days, the sadness of my mom's circumstances interfered with the fun of formulating wedding plans.

I guess staying busy kept the enormity of my circumstances at bay. Every day of summer was spent on task preparing for two tearful life milestones, albeit tears of different genres. I was too industrious to comprehend what the future held as two of my primary and defining roles were entering transformation at the same moment. My role as Bonnie's mother was about to change, and my role as Joan's daughter was about to expire.

Sadly, this last month long hospital stay was unlike the previous visits which seemed to give Joan a shot in the arm. This stay was not good for her health. They put her in a wheel chair to keep her from falling. Mom hated the wheelchair. They forced this rubber lap guard, called a buddy, under the arms of the wheelchair, so she was prevented from escaping out of the chair. One day, I saw a big, strong, crazed woman lean forward, grasp the buddy, and walk down the hall with her wheelchair out behind her like a huge metal frame with wheels mounted on her ass. I bet Joan would have done that if she could. Mom's legs didn't do well not moving, and they began to swell. An order for support hose was the answer. The glucose in the IV caused her sugar levels to become abnormal. An order for diabetic medicine was the answer. An open wound at her tailbone developed from malnourishment. Bandaging was applied. Mom developed a highly contagious diarrhea sickness commonly found in hospital settings. Isolation was necessary. We had to put protective gear on before entering her room. The longer she stayed, the more problems arose. She was lost, and the quality of her life was fiercely lacking. As for the electroconvulsive therapy, if you visited right after a session, she was dazed and confused. If you visited the next day, the effect was gone. If you timed it just right, perhaps the evening of an ECT day, you experienced a limited conversation. Scott was privileged to partake in one such exchange of dialogue. In the end, he believed the ECT was worthwhile for the simple fact that he got to enjoy one last evening of conversation and improved clarity with his mom before she left us for good. I never timed it right.

The doctor did not witness enough improvement in Joan's mental health to warrant the continuation of the expensive and partly experimental electroconvulsive therapy. He quit the treatment even before the prescribed plan was completed. I must admit I was relieved. I didn't feel good at all about her time in the hospital. We had so little control of her life there. She appeared oblivious to her surroundings, but how did we really know? If she could communicate, she may have screamed, "Get me out of here!" She was discharged for the last time. It was time to discuss Hospice. I think we were all ready for this last step. Fortunately, Country Gardens was open to the idea of Mom staying with them in her comfortable room for the end of her life with that added support of a Hospice team.

We all met with the Hospice team the day after Mom came home from the hospital. Mom, Scott, a Hospice nurse, a Hospice chaplain, the Hospice director, the Country Gardens director, the Country Gardens nurse, and I all sat in a circle in Joan's room. It was July 14. We discussed the procedures of Hospice care. Mom had a living will, and resuscitation measures were clearly defined as not her wishes. We received the little, blue Hospice booklet explaining the natural death process. They ordered a hospital bed, a wheel chair, and oxygen tanks to be delivered the next day. The Hospice nurse took Joan off all medications except for the anxiety drugs, pain meds, and sedatives. This was my first experience with this service, and I must say Scott and I were impressed with the organization and clarity of the whole Hospice team. Again, Scott phoned Mark with each step to keep him in the loop.

Steve and I removed Mom's bed the next day when her hospital bed arrived at Country Gardens. The new bed came with great new technology, an air mattress with columns of chambers hooked up to a pump that was constantly inflating and deflating sections at a time to decrease the chances of bed sores. A strange thing happened when we made up Mom's new bed. She crawled in it and stayed there. The fear of her falling was thankfully diminished as she put up camp in her new bed. It might have been the sedative medication, her weakness from loss of weight, or maybe even the comfort of those rising and falling air chambers, but I think it was her decision to get in that comfortable bed and die.

I went back to visiting with her every day now that she was so close, close to my house again, close to death. She was incredibly thin. I tried to get her to eat at lunchtime. She had begun the habit of packing any food I put in her mouth into her cheeks like a chipmunk. Little food went down the esophagus, and if it did, she often choked. The assisted living kitchen staff was pureeing her food which helped somewhat. I helped her walk to her little kitchen table. She would open her mouth for me to put in a spoonful. It took such energy and effort for her to swallow that a ten-bite lunch could take an hour. It was clear that her interest in nourishment was over. The labor and process of getting food in my mom brought up a recollection from my youth. I rescued a baby bird once and kind of force-fed it. I didn't know if I overfed it or underfed it, but the bird died.

After lunch, Joan would crawl back in her bed. I was changing her diapers often and continuing to help her in the shower. I just thought it must feel awful to not get cleaned up regularly. Her diarrhea was still prevalent. The wound at her tailbone was still unhealed. Even though the staff at Country Gardens and the Hospice nurses would clean her up, they weren't there as often as she needed, or they weren't as thorough and gentle as her daughter. Somehow you manage, knowing that mother would do the same for daughter if the roles were reversed. Dignity was a factor. There was something offensive about strangers seeing my mom naked. I tried to keep her dignity intact. You know, do unto others.

For three weeks life carried on like this, Joan in the bed, Joan hardly eating, Joan getting a ride around the building in her new wheel chair, Joan sleeping a lot, Joan getting cleaned up. Country Gardens kept a good watch, and Hospice nurses checked in two or three times a week. Scott and I visited at different times of the day, he in the evenings, but we still talked to each other constantly. From the beginning, we often shared with each other our deepest thoughts concerning Mom's situation. Nothing was off limits. We worked through our feelings of guilt when we were tired and just wanted it all to end. We talked about the speed of Mom's deterioration and how sad it was, how quickly she declined. Then, we'd do an about face and realize it was a blessing, her quick decline. I knew of people whose parents with Alzheimer's spent years in a vegetative state. The visits to their parents dwindled as time went by. Their medical bills ballooned. We were able to maintain a constant involvement with the end of our mom's life. She would have wanted it to end quickly, and maybe she did have some control over the situation.

The director at Country Gardens, Mary Beth, started calling me and telling me Mom looked close. She thought it would be soon. I spent a great deal of time sitting by her bed on a deathwatch. Throughout it all, the family bond was strong and effective. My brother and I could count on each other. My husband and children were a source of great strength as they supported me emotionally. Steve was always ready to help out in any way he could. The staff at the hospital, at Hospice, and at Country Gardens all provided information and procedures. But someone who also helped keep me sane was someone not a part of my family, nor employed by a geriatric health organization, my best girlfriend, Lea Anne, my loyal pal in life. I don't know what I would have done without her.

Chapter 13 The Friend

I knew of Lea Anne in high school, but we were not in the same crowd. I remember the first time our eyes met. While walking in opposite directions down the congested hallways, the misbehaving wire in my spiral notebook snagged her sweater. She gave me one of the biggest eat shit looks I had ever received. We met again under different circumstances the summer after high school graduation. I had a new boyfriend, and he was good friends with her boyfriend. We double dated a few times. It turned out Lea Anne and I were suited more to each other than to either of our young love boyfriends. We eventually dumped them and kept each other.

We started hanging out when our boyfriends had other things to do. That meant we hit all the local bars on their "drink special" nights. Tuesday was Nickel Night at Greene's. Wednesday was Zoo Night at the Warehouse where three dollars at the door got you a big red cup for free drinks all night. Thursday was three for one at Harlow's. Cheap drinks, checking out the man scene, and dancing to "Funky Town" filled our nights for a couple of years. Then, I met Steve. Lea Anne was there. She gave me a bridal shower. We cried in our cocktails when I moved to Canada. She was the maid of honor at my wedding. We hugged upon my return to the states.

Our lives progressed along unlike paths, however. Steve and I started a family. Lea Anne finished her dental hygiene training and led the Mary Tyler Moore lifestyle. She bought a condominium with her sister, worked, traveled, and dated. She came to visit occasionally, adorned in her stylish outfits, bringing my children some cool new toy or book. I met her at the door with my sweat pants and ponytail. I was a suburban housewife. She wasn't. We still kept in touch but didn't see as much of each other.

Lea Anne got married the year Steve and I celebrated our tenth anniversary. I was so happy to give her a wedding shower. She had given and attended so many on my behalf. It didn't seem fair. Phil was her elementary school sweetheart. In high school he moved to a neighboring town, and they lost touch for years. When they hooked up this time, it was for good. We all went out together on occasion, and we enjoyed each other's company. Lea Anne and I had long replaced the nightclub scene with outings to local home tours, art festivals, and craft shows when we could. But I was still wrapped up in ballet lessons, karate lessons, soccer and baseball, Easter egg hunts and Halloween costumes, homework and birthday parties. Our life was our kids. Lea Anne and Phil chose not to have any children.

About the time my kids decided friends were more fun than family on Friday nights, the Friday night phone call tradition began. Lea Anne and Phil lived about an hour away from our suburb in a more rural setting, so getting together often was rather difficult. Therefore, every Friday night around six o'clock, Lea Anne and I pour a glass of wine and pick up the phone. We talk about our week. We talk about what is happening in the outside world. We share our personal worlds with each other. We give each other the gift of undivided attention, really listening. We provide counsel only when necessary. It is our therapy. Sometimes, our weeks are so full; the discussions go on for hours and multiple refills to the wine glass.

Lea Anne and I like to have a life observation we find humorous ready to share each week. Once, on a drive to Florida, Steve and I were fully entertained by the billboards. I would be ready to share our amusement with Lea Anne on the next Friday conversation. On one side of the highway we read, "We Bare All! Truckers welcome! Full nudity! Adult toys and DVDs!" On the other side of the highway we read, "Jesus Saves! Let Jesus pay your toll! Let's meet at my house on Sunday before the game! – God." I mentioned my frustration with these extreme values to Steve and questioned the need in life for either proposition. "Isn't there a middle road?" I asked him.

He answered, "How about Bare All for Jesus."

Lea Anne and I discuss current events. It helps that we usually share similar viewpoints when it comes to politics and religion. I'd keep her up to date on the latest antics on the Colbert Report, as Stephen Colbert was one of my favorite funny guys. Lea Anne loved to write down the sayings on church marquees she found amusing. She shared them with me. "If God has a refrigerator, would your picture be on it? The best vitamin for Christians is B-1. Without the bread of life, you're toast." Those were some of her favorites. During the time the Baptists were debating their controversy of whether or not to allow women to become ministers, we had some choice words to say. I told her, "I guess the Baptist preacher man has come up with yet one more purpose for that omnipotent penis, an antenna to God." We laughed.

Lea Anne and I discuss women's issues quite often. I hated the mail that was addressed to Mrs. (fill in the husband's name here). Married women have a name; we aren't an appendage of our husband. My mom had shared with me a similar frustration on her job because so many elderly women lacked financial knowledge. These women were lost in the bank after the death of their husbands. The number of teenage girls becoming pregnant appalled Lea Anne. What happened to the women's movement? Where was the passion for equality displayed in the seventies? Even with all our advancements, sexism doesn't appear to be leaving society any time soon. Lea Anne told me about a dentist she once worked for who instructed the hygienists to allow him to remove all female patients' spit bibs at the conclusion of the dental exam. He wanted to be the one to reveal what endowment lay underneath. Absurd. After passing by a Hooter's billboard, I shared with Lea Anne my idea to open up a restaurant called Woody's. The advertising mascot would be a woodpecker bird with an oversized beak. The male waiters would be shirtless and wear tight shorts depicting a woodpecker's head in the crotch area, emphasizing their packages in the confines of a bright yellow beak. They would serve cucumber sandwiches, a variety of salads, and provide a large wine assortment. We liked to try out our comic abilities on each other.

Lea Anne and I discuss other problems we see with society. We sympathized with my good friend who taught kindergarten and happened to be gay. She won teacher of the year, yet our principal told her not to bring her partner of twenty years to the awards night celebration. It wouldn't look good. We complained about the demise of small town America, quaint old downtowns boarding up their storefronts because of another Wal-Mart moving in at Exit Ten. We questioned if people would remain as complacent and quiet if white teenage boys instead of black teenage boys were being shot and killed every night in South Side Atlanta. We talked about warped priorities. Why did so many athletes make astronomical salaries while so many in our country suffered in poverty? We feared for the emotional well being of the soldiers coming home from the Middle East. A few of them were killing their wives at a nearby army post's family quarters. We wondered if the little Chinese children who were making the latest plastic toy for our American children to play with wanted to play with the toy too. Did they get to take just one home? We thought people who wanted to keep evolution out of our textbooks should just look at my dog's face after a bath. He's a seal! We discussed the killings by the drug cartel in the town in Mexico near the US border. I figured crime would greatly decrease if America legalized and regulated drugs. The dealers would be out of a job. Girls wouldn't have to sell their bodies for a fix. Instead of spending money on prisons, we could provide drug users with counseling and job training. We were frustrated with the sad situation of illegal immigrants. I knew of a young man who was robbed but scared to report it because he was undocumented. Patriotic Americans seem fine with the atrocities immigrants experience in the USA. How quickly they forget. It makes me think about the Eagles song, "The Last Resort." I always loved that song. "We satisfy our endless needs/and justify our bloody deeds/In the name of destiny/and in the name of God."

I often question the role of ideology in this world. I think a lot about it. One cause that I support passionately is a woman's right to choose. I don't understand how anyone can believe a man in a black robe, who has never experienced childbirth, who lives a thousand miles away, who doesn't know me, hasn't even met me, should have any say in my decision making process on probably the most important choice of my life. And I do support the right to life, a child's right to a healthy life. That includes a life where the child is wanted, where the child will have a family who will provide support, love, and care. And women who make this choice might need our help. It seems strange to me that the same folks who oppose abortion because it's inhumane are usually the same folks who support less socialized government to help the poor, who support wars that destroy innocent life, who support gun ownership which often ends up in tragedy, and who support capital punishment which is breaking one of the commandments. Isn't this value system inconsistent? An embryo or fetus must never die, a person, well that's fine in some cases. So the pro-lifer counsels the poor and lonely girl to keep her baby. The pro-lifer votes in to office the compassionate conservatives. Now that wee, precious babe born in poverty to the single mom is facing a struggle without programs such as Head Start. With fewer food stamps, the mom has to work overtime at her minimum wage job. The funding for after school programs has been cut, and the child is hungry, frustrated, and alone every afternoon. Gang life is ready to fill the void. The precious babe resorts to crime. He gets a gun from a buddy, uses it, and ends up in prison. He's now on death row, and the right to lifers are picketing outside his cell with signs that say death to criminals. WTF? I don't understand. Maybe my beliefs are just as inconsistent. I cry when baby seals are clubbed, yet I support safe, legal abortion. It's confusing isn't it? It's hard to find moderation in this issue. The pro-life movement's answer is adoption, a lovely idea. We have more than 14,000 children in foster care in the state of Georgia alone. Where are all the adoptive parents? How about teaching more birth control information in schools? That's a start. Abstinence only is a joke. It's just what I think about it all, the whole pro-choice situation and the whole liberal-conservative situation, and lots of other people think differently than me, about half our country actually.

Anyway, during the Friday night conversations, Lea Anne and I don't always talk about such deep stuff. We celebrate our successes in life too. We provide each other with kudos over our accomplishments, no matter how trivial. We both are engaged in very busy lives. Lea Anne has her career but also manages the office work of her husband's business, a big job. I always seem to be back in school working on some degree or painting a house or planning an event for someone in the family. We sometimes compete in our bragging tales of how many errands we can complete on a Saturday. "I have to go to the bank to open an IRA, stop by the post office to mail some cards to Canada, pick up our prescriptions at the pharmacy, return some books to the library, sew and hang these dining room curtains that have been sitting here for a week, and go to the grocery store tomorrow," I'd say.

"That's a lot. I'm visiting Phil's mom in the hospital, taking back a sweater to Macy's, going by the tag office for a new license plate, picking up the dry cleaning, picking up a ring that was re-sized at the jewelers, fetching Maggie's medicine at the vet's office, and getting a haircut tomorrow," she replied.

Sometimes, things were so busy in our lives; we wondered if we had it right. We wondered what it would feel like to quit our jobs, let everything go, live in a trailer in the woods, and drink beer on the porch every day. Lea Anne was always more sure than I was that we had it right. Sometimes, I didn't know.

We discuss books a lot. We evolved from our youthful practice of reading Sidney Sheldon tales or romance novels with the long haired, muscular men on the covers to more sophisticated reading. Lea Anne chose titles from the newspaper reviews, and I chose titles from Oprah's book club list. We traded worthy reads. She went through a nonfiction phase, and I went through a high school required reading phase. Too many times I only read the Cliff Notes in those days. We both loved John Irving novels. Of course, our favorite was *Cider House Rules*.

Through the years on Friday nights, however, our most time consuming topic has been our families. Lea Anne listened to my woes as I balanced divorced parents and holidays. I listened to her talk about her father's losing battle with cancer. Sometimes, we talked about my strained relationship with my brother Mark. Sometimes, we talked about her strained relationship with her sister Karen. Our husbands' family dramas provided plenty of discussion too. Of course, Lea Anne listened to all the trials and triumphs of Bonnie and Lee as they grew up. The opportunity to work through any family issue with someone who shares no genetic similarity is invaluable to us both. I realize that now, Mom, the nourishment you received from your girlfriends helped get you through life.

Friday night is best friend time. It takes something big to cancel out the Friday night phone call, sometimes to the dismay of our husbands. Those weekly conversations with Lea Anne during Joan's demise were an important strategy for working through my anxiety. I learned in one of my psychology classes that being responsible for the welfare of the mentally ill or the physically handicapped is extremely stressful on a caregiver, and having a support system in place is crucial. Lea Anne was a big part of my support system. The Friday night ear, always ready to listen, fulfilling that basic need in us all just to be heard, that was a beautiful thing.

Our friendship did go beyond our phone call routine. When Bonnie and Lee were almost grown and old enough to manage without Mom and Dad for a long weekend, Steve and I started going on short trips with Lea Anne and Phil. Grandma would stay at the house to provide some supervision. My mother taught me to make time in life for good friends and great getaways. She loved supporting my relationship with Lea Anne and loved keeping up with Lea Anne's life too. So about once a year, Lea Anne, Phil, Steve, and I went to destinations like Asheville, North Carolina, New Orleans, or Cumberland Island, Georgia. We took turns picking a destination. One of the most memorable trips was the one Steve planned for us all, a houseboat excursion on the Suwannee River.

The guys fished. Lea Anne and I divided our time between reading and chatting. We all took turns steering the boat up the wide and lazy river, a true Southern beauty. Beautiful flora and fauna appeared at every turn.

Moss draped trees lined the slow moving black water. Large sturgeons, up to eight feet in length, were hurling themselves into the air and reentering the water with a monumental splash. While swimming by the banks, we could hear and see the munching of manatees feeding on the water lettuce. Steve swam down and got close enough to touch them. We rowed to shore in the dinghy to visit the brilliant, turquoise waters of the natural springs that fed the river. We witnessed the watercolor sky at day's end twice, both over our heads and under our chins as a reflection in the water. The sense of relaxation found in this special place was unmatched. Then, it got dark.

Upon retiring, we heard this strange, low, grinding sound coming from the boat. Steve turned on his flashlight. Phil turned on his flashlight. There were about a hundred three-inch cockroaches darting all over the houseboat! They were on our beds, on our pillows, on the floor, everywhere! I started screaming. This scene, straight from a horror show, totally corrupted my picturesque image of the river by light. I remember being balled up in fetal position with the sheet over my head in a constant wiggle movement to keep them at bay just waiting for the sun to come up and save us. Never was a night longer than that one.

Steve received much heckling from us for choosing and planning this voyage. We banned him from any further trip planning. He smiled through it all. For him, the roaches didn't diminish the memories of peace and beauty that transpired during the light hours. Steve still recalls this trip as his favorite. The rest of us shudder when we hear the melody that begins, "Way down upon the Suwannee River."

As far as really close friends go, Lea Anne and I laugh at our low number, one each. I was always amazed and impressed with the number of friends my mom kept up with throughout her life. But with full time work and family obligations, I never really had the time or the desire for additional best friends. Lea Anne was it. I have enjoyed camaraderie with many of my former neighbors, especially those from the house we lived in for eighteen years, the house where my children grew up. We had some great neighborhood parties as we lived in a new development, and most of the buyers were young with small children like us. But I rarely see any of those friends anymore. I have enjoyed camaraderie with fellow education coworkers through the years, but rarely did those relationships carry over into personal time. There is something healthy about separating work and home life. I have enjoyed camaraderie with a few friends from my youth. There were occasional phone calls, Christmas cards, a summer luncheon, and high school reunions. However, one relationship I put a little more effort in staying connected with was the one I had with Fran.

Fran and I had lost touch for many years. But strangely enough, we found ourselves living about a mile away from each other at a time when we could rekindle our friendship. Her kids were high school ages like mine were when we discovered how close we were. On a few summer late afternoons, I found myself at Fran's house for happy hour. I'd sit at her kitchen table and regress back to the habits we shared in our youth, drinking beer and smoking cigarettes. I think the allure of hooting and hollering with a Miller Lite in one hand and a Benson and Hedges Light in the other never completely leaves those who embraced that lifestyle when they were young.

Fran made me laugh in my youth and when we found each other again. While visiting one night, I was listening to Fran discuss the frustrations of dealing with her own aging mother's health problems. Fran was experiencing the stress of being the primary caregiver years before me. She blurted out, "Christ on a pony, I've taken my mother to every doctor from asshole to shoe sole, and still there's no relief." Fran had a way with words.

I saw her on Ash Wednesday and asked her why she didn't have the smudge on her forehead. Her husband answered for her. "She didn't make it to church. No big deal, Fran will just snuff out the last cigarette of the day on her forehead. I told her I'd help her get to church when they celebrated Thong Thursday instead of Ash Wednesday." He had a way with words too. He wasn't a Catholic.

For a little while, the appeal of the past kept us going. We rehashed some of our old, crazy days. We shook our heads at how out of it our parents were. We shook our heads over our own young stupidity. We roared with laughter at so many memories. We caught up on the gossip of some of the high school folks we had run into over the years.

But after a while, our visits dwindled, the pull of old time partying just wasn't the same. Fran and I returned to occasional phone calls, Christmas cards, a summer luncheon, and high school reunions. But Fran is an old friend that I can count on to attend my daughter's wedding and my mother's funeral. I attended both her parents' funerals. I hope to go to her daughter's wedding one day. Who knows, I may even laugh at her kitchen table again in the future.

Chapter 14   The Death

Mom's eyes became so blue that weekend. She was skin, bone, white hair, and blue eyes. Somehow, though, I thought she looked beautiful. My only experience with her version of thinness was through photographs in history books depicting the Holocaust. Every bone was prominent. I was able to completely encircle her collarbone with my thumb and pointer finger with only her skin between my fingertips as they met behind the clavicle, making an okay sign. She wasn't okay though. She was dying.

The Country Gardens director Mary Beth phoned Hospice and me very early on Saturday morning, the fourth of August. Joan was demonstrating some difficulty breathing. I phoned Scott as he had been with Mom the night before for quite some time. We reluctantly shared views on how much longer we thought she would hold on. I headed over to Country Gardens. The weekend Hospice nurse, Pouran, arrived shortly after. She was the nurse that had met Mom at the initial introductory meeting three weeks prior and hadn't seen Joan since. She was a little surprised at the difference in her health in such a short time. The Joan she first met was walking around, still displaying bright eyes. This Joan was lying on her back, eyes rolling at times, legs moving up and down rhythmically under the covers. Pouran looked her over and took her vital signs. She predicted life expectancy of a couple of days. She showed Mary Beth and me how to use the oxygen machine to help Mom breathe less laboriously. She was concerned about Mom choking, so she ordered NBM, nothing by mouth. She ordered Mom's sedative medicine to come in a lotion to rub on her arms. She explained what was happening with Joan's body, the process of shutting down. Her pulse, blood pressure, and body temperature readings were all pointing to the end. She thought Mom looked serene, and the oxygen and sedative would allow her to pass peacefully. I liked this nurse. Pouran was in her last year of medical school, preparing to be a doctor. She was knowledgeable and kind.

After Pouran left, I sat with Mom and cried. It seemed so cruel to follow the rule of nothing by mouth. I bet Joan was thirsty. I called Steve, and he said he was on his way over. I talked to Mom and rubbed her head as she slept. I watched the many expressions on her face changing from smiles to frowns, her eyebrows arching up as if surprised. I remember so clearly holding my infants, mesmerized by the changing expressions on their faces while they slept. I couldn't help but notice the ironic similarity. Here I was, able to behold a sleeping, final face, perhaps rewinding a life, so similar to beholding a sleeping, fresh face, perhaps previewing the life ahead.

Joan's peacefulness was sometimes interrupted by a jolt of wakefulness, her eyes open, legs moving up and down, and jaw flying back and forth. When her agitation returned, the bedside chair became more uncomfortable. Steve suggested I tell her not to fight and tell her all would be fine. He had arrived and brought strength and wisdom with him.

Her frustration increased when she was aware of the oxygen tube placed in her nose. She pawed at that apparatus, scowling. We only kept it in when she was restful or sleeping. The tubes in her nose reminded me of the time I was watching a soap opera on a summer day when I was of high school age. My mom hated soap operas. She thought all that sleeping around was disgraceful. I was watching a hospital scene with a dying woman on the bed. She had oxygen tubes in her nose. My mom walked by and quietly stated, "Up your nose with a rubber hose." During that overly dramatic, somber TV moment, we broke out in laughter. I was missing our silliness already. Steve and I shared this long day alone with Joan, reminiscing and just being present.

I didn't realize then how important that day alone with Joan was. I was given the time to proceed through a stage of acceptance. I was allowed one last quiet day before the chaos set in, and the business of dying materialized. Precious. I sat next to her and reviewed my life with this woman. I thought about the shortcomings and the treasures of our relationship. The treasures shone through. The shortcomings paled. I was thankful for that tipping of the balance to the positive side. I was thankful that throughout my adult life I was able to pay tribute to and celebrate with this exceptional lady. I chose to remember the good times, the invaluable knowledge she imparted, and the example she led. I was lucky to have her as my role model. I attempted to forgive and forget the troubled youth years. With maturity, I realized she was in her own world of pain during those years, making proper parenting difficult. We never really talked with any psychological depth about my misbehaving adolescence. Should we have? I don't know. Is ignoring the past or pretending something never happened ever healthy? She watched me parent my teenage children differently and complimented me on the job I was doing. Was that her form of an apology? Forgiveness is a difficult concept to embrace, and I'm not sure I ever completely succeeded. Forgiveness was evident in my actions but not always evident in my mind. Is that the best we can do? People talk a lot about forgiving and forgetting. People talk a lot about regrets too. I was thankful I had no regrets, none. We left her at ten o'clock that night, wondering what the next day would bring.

Sunday morning, I woke up at 5:30 and got up to get ready to head over to Country Gardens. When I walked into Joan's room, she was sitting up, looking radiant. Her eyes were bright, and her color was good. She mouthed "hello" to me and attempted a smile that morning. I managed to get her up out of the bed and into the shower, supporting her one hundred percent. She was pretty light in her skeletal state. I put her in fresh pajamas. She got back in the bed. I dipped her toothbrush into mouthwash and brushed her teeth. I brushed her hair. I soaked her fingernails in soapy water and removed the crud out from under them with her nail file. She was going to have visitors.

Bonnie and a girlfriend of hers visited that afternoon. It was difficult for me to see Bonnie's tears. Scott and Diana came over in the afternoon. Steve was by my side most of the time. We all congregated in Joan's room and tried to make each other feel better by talking about funny stuff. Mary Beth was always close at hand to see if we needed anything. She checked on our well being as much as she had been checking on Joan's the last few weeks. As the day wore on, Mom wore out. It was Scott and Diana's wedding anniversary, so they left to go out for a nice dinner at a close by restaurant. When they returned, Steve and I went home. Scott and Diana stayed with Joan until midnight. The night nurse predicted correctly that she would still be there in the morning. I remembered hearing that people only lasted three days without water. The next day would be day three of nothing by mouth.

Monday was supposed to be my first day back to work; planning days had begun for the new school year. I called the secretary to let her know what was going on and that I didn't know when I would be able to return to work. Missing work was foreign to me. My mother taught me to follow the puritan work ethic, to show up no matter what and not let down any coworkers. But Mom dying trumped the puritan work ethic. Steve also called his office to explain the circumstances and his decision to stay with me. He received total support. We arrived at Country Gardens early in the morning.

Mom looked tired, and the brightness present Sunday morning had dimmed. She had a busy day in store despite her appearance. I phoned the kids, and they made plans to come over. A chaplain we had never met from Hospice came for a visit. No tranquility or insight entered my soul from the words or prayers of that chaplain. She had never met Joan before; she was a stranger. When she was explaining to me about what my mom was going through, I wanted to ask her how she knew what my mom was going through. I spent forty-six years listening to this woman. I had been taking care of her for the last few years, daily care for quite some time. I think I had a better handle on what my mom was going through than some woman who felt she was closer to God because she took a training course. What was meant as a ritual to bring peace to a family just brought me aggravation. Steve tried to moderate my resentment by explaining that the chaplain was only trying to help. Steve was my constant voice of reason.

The minister from the church my mom attended came for a visit. I felt better about this one. She really did know my mom, and her words were comforting. She sensed my needs and acted accordingly, a sign of good counsel. Two of my colleagues came to see us. They had never met my mom before, and I wished they were meeting her under different circumstances. I wished they were meeting the Joan of years past. I was always proud to introduce my kind and funny mom to any of my acquaintances. Scott arrived and let me know that he had notified Mark in Texas to tell him to get to Georgia quickly. Bonnie and Joe and Lee arrived. For a short time the room was overcrowded with guests, too crowded. Eventually, non-family members said their goodbyes, and the family stayed. At one point, everyone except Bonnie and Lee left the room so the grandchildren could have some alone time with their beloved Grandma. This was the Grandma who came to every birthday party, the grandma who went to soccer games and dance recitals, the grandma who came over when Mommy and Daddy wanted a date night, the grandma who watched them open presents from Santa, and the grandma who made them root beer floats on New Year's Eve. I mentioned to Bonnie and Lee that now was the time to tell her anything they needed to tell her.

Mom appeared rather oblivious to all the commotion of the day. That evening, I called Pouran to let her know Joan was still with us and that I was concerned about the practice of nothing by mouth for such a long time. I wondered what sort of suffering went along with this practice. Was it ethical? I wanted another visit by a medical person. We hadn't seen one since Saturday. Pouran said the weekday nurse would be there in the morning. I had met Jennifer a few times in the last three weeks, and I liked her as well. Pouran told me I could give Joan some water. I gave Mom a drink by holding my finger over the end of a half-filled straw and releasing the water between her lips. She turned her head so slowly toward me and opened her mouth like a baby bird for some more. My soul ached with sorrow at that action of despondency.

Monday was another late night bedtime followed by another early morning the next day. I had been sleeping fitfully every night for a while, wondering if my mom would be breathing the next morning. Tuesday, the seventh of August would put an end to that sickening nighttime sensation. Steve and I arrived at Country Gardens early in the morning. Mom was the color of ash. The nurse Jennifer arrived soon after, immediately recognizing the need to hasten Joan's journey to the other side. She explained the role of morphine at this point. Mark, Scott, and Diana walked into the room. Mark hadn't seen Mom since June. I'm sure Scott tried to prepare him for what he was about to walk into, but I'm not sure that preparation is possible. Mark did very well. He thanked her for waiting until he got there. That was quite a gift she gave Mark, waiting to die until he arrived. I could hear her. "I have three children, not two. I'm not going anywhere until they are all here." We all discussed the need for something, morphine being the something, according to Jennifer. Steve wanted to wait to begin the administering until he spoke with Bonnie, to offer her the choice of being present. Bonnie and Joe had slept over the night before, and they were just waking up back at the house. Bonnie told her dad to wait. They would be right over. Lee had already gone to work for the day, his goodbyes the day before would have to suffice.

There we were, gathered around our mom's bed, her three children, Scott, Mark, and Candy. Steve, Diana, Bonnie and Joe formed the outer circle, close behind us. We told Mom to go to the arms of her parents. We told her we would all be fine. We told her we would miss her. We told her it was okay to let go. We each took a turn to express our personal final thoughts to our mom. I thanked her for being such a wonderful mom. I told her I was sorry for all the nagging I had done in the last couple of years, sorry for making her do things she didn't want to do, and sorry that my actions made her mad at me. I know the real Joan would have thanked me for all I took on with her house and her care. I know the real Joan would have been appreciative. I still felt the need to apologize before I told her I loved her.

We stepped aside when the nurse put the morphine under Mom's tongue. Joan lacked muscle or fat tissue for injections. We stared at her. She stared back. Scott pointed to a tear that was slowly rolling out of her fading blue eye. I hadn't seen a tear fall from her eye in the last six months. The drugs she was on kept emotions at bay. We all cried. We talked about memories. We remembered Mom singing "You Are My Sunshine" to us as kids. Steve suggested we all sing the song to her. We did, complete with harmony, the way she liked. Mom's breathing was labored, so the nurse gave her some more morphine. We rubbed her hands and arms and head. We waited.

At 11:01 a.m., she took a big breath and then silently stopped breathing. All that could be heard in her Country Gardens apartment was the sniffling of her family. The personal thoughts that must have been running through each of our heads were interrupted at 11:04 when she inhaled again as if fighting for breath. She resumed her labored inhalation and exhalation. We all looked at the nurse. Jennifer explained to us that this sometimes happens. We knew Mom didn't want to leave us all. There she was, with her three kids around her, and she didn't want it to end. She tricked us again at 11:10. She took a deep breath, let it go as a sigh, and became still once more. Four minutes went by this time. We were even beginning to stir and murmur when Joan gave us the jolt of our lives. She sounded like she was exploding out of the swimming pool, winning the hold your breath under water the longest contest. She wouldn't give in without a fight. Jennifer told us she had never seen this before, resuming breathing for a second time after four minutes of stillness. We told her Joan was one stubborn lady. The room's aura held on to and embraced the sadness, but bits of comic relief, disbelief, frustration, and mostly discomfort swirled through the air. At 11:21, the sigh that left Joan's body was truly her last. I whispered my final goodbye and left the room.

Chapter 15   The Arrangements

I didn't want to be in the room with her like that. I had to sign some papers with Jennifer and Mary Beth. They called the cremation society to come pick up the body. The smokers among us went to the parking lot. I thought about how good a cigarette would taste right then if I still smoked. My brothers called our father to tell him the news. Steve called Lee. We waited in a sitting area with the assisted living residents coming by for a chat now and then, oblivious to the recent events. Their confusion worked well as protection in times like these. In fact, the truck that pulled up to the front door with the words Cremation Society of the South written boldly on the side panel didn't even initiate a look of bewilderment or a questioning glance from any of the residents rocking away on the front porch.

The men who came to shake our hands and take our mom's body provided us with a much-needed giggle. It was just too predictable. One was very tall and lanky, and the other was short and stout. Their suits were ill fitted, and we couldn't decide if their hair was a wig or just a bad dye job. Each generation had a comparison, Laurel and Hardy, Abbot and Costello, or the Roxbury Guys, Steve and Doug Butabi. Their stereotypical appearance created a brief, enjoyable diversion.

With everything taken care of at Country Gardens, we hugged Jennifer, Mary Beth, and the ladies who watched over my mom for the last year. We told them we would come back later throughout the week to clean out Joan's room and to give them information on her service arrangements. We all went out to lunch. I ordered a glass of wine. I hadn't had anything to drink in the last week as all my time was spent at Joan's bedside. It was the first of many that day for me. When we left the restaurant, we all headed to our house to continue bonding as the children and family of deceased Joan.

Bonnie and Joe returned to their home fairly early. They had a two-hour drive. I promised to call when arrangements were made, so they could organize another trip back. Steve called his family in Canada. Mark called his girlfriend in Texas. I called Lea Anne and described the day's events to her. She listened. I praised the experience of being present at my mom's death. Lea Anne and I had talked about the benefits of assisted suicide in a past Friday night conversation. The contrast between that beautiful passing surrounded by loved ones, my mom able to see our faces, hear our voices, feel our touch, to slipping away alone in a vacant and dark room only strengthened my belief in the compassionate practice of choosing the right time to die. How many Hospice nurses know this truth and provide the right amount of morphine while the patient is surrounded by family? Why can't this be an accepted and legal choice? What if Mom slipped away in the night? I know I would have felt frustratingly incomplete, guilty, and even more hurt.

For the rest of the evening, Scott, Mark, and I sat in the basement talking about immediate plans and long ago memories with beer and wine in hand. Diana drove my brothers home late that night. Steve listened to me babble on and on until we fell asleep. The alcohol erased the image of my mom's lifeless body until one o'clock in the morning when it returned accompanied by a headache. Certain images were imprinting themselves in my brain during my wakeful states of emotional exhaustion. Three were prominent. The first image was of Joan on Sunday morning attempting a smile and mouthing "hello." The second image was her head turning toward my water filled straw, desperately opening her mouth for a drop. The third image was the tear that rolled down her face moments before her final breath. Young and vibrant Joan was mingling with old and tired Joan in my distressed dream state that night.

Wednesday, the eighth of August was a day of responsible errands. Steve drove Scott, Mark, and me to them all. He was our chauffeur and our man of good judgment. We had a morning appointment at the cremation society to pick out an urn. We met with Jessica and began the paperwork. The mood was light, and Mom's sense of humor was emitting from us all. We asked Jessica what the little urns that looked like salt and pepper shakers were for. She explained that some families like to share the remains. We laughed about fighting over a leg or an arm. Jessica took this moment to let us know her nickname, Deathica. She predicted correctly we would appreciate her sense of humor, as would Joan. Her license plate displayed the name, and we had to go see her car on our way out. We left with the purchase of a plain urn meant for burial. I wanted to bury Mom's ashes in the beautiful, old cemetery on Grand Island, NY where her parents were buried. Scott chose the brass nameplate depicting a nature scene. We all agreed. Steve suggested we have "You Are My Sunshine" engraved under her name. So we did.

Our afternoon appointment was with Mom's pastor at the Methodist Church. She wanted to discuss the essence of Joan and plan for the memorial service. She was a fabulous lady and guided us with ease through the difficult process of determining how the service should flow. We all agreed on a celebration of life with the focus on remembering Joan. We all agreed that we could each get up, approach the altar, and speak to the congregation about our mom. As difficult as that would be for some people, none of us exhibited a hint of hesitation or doubt in our abilities. We narrowed down the essence of Joan into three categories, her gift of wit, her display of kindness, and her love of the arts. Scott was going to begin by acknowledging her wit. I would present next by celebrating her kindness. Mark would portray her love of the arts. We chose music pieces and readings. We devised a time-line and wrote down our to-do lists. The service was set for Saturday at eleven in the morning. I shed some tears during this appointment. Joan's essence was hard to talk about in the past tense.

We went back to the house and ordered pizza. After supper, Scott and Mark went back to Scott's house. This was the evening that I dedicated to phoning all my mom's friends. She had so many, and I knew most of them. I was very familiar with Joan's address book. I had helped Mom in recent years with her Christmas Cards. I always enjoyed reading the basket full of cards my mom acquired at Christmas time. I made it a point to look through her cards with her every year since I moved away from home. She would take this opportunity to let me know what was going on in each of the lives of her friends. Giving them the news was going to be heartbreaking.

I began each conversation the same. I told them who I was, and then I told them the news. I repeated this about twenty times and over great distances that night. No matter how I worded it, Joan has passed, Joan has died, Joan is gone, I couldn't get the words out without choking and crying as each lady listened on the other end of the line. Some things aren't easier with repetition. Their responses were as varied as the ladies themselves. Some of them immediately stated it was a blessing. Some of them cried. Some of them couldn't believe that Joan's spirit was extinguished so quickly. Some had just sent her a card. Some refused to have contact with her the last year because she just wasn't the same old Joan. But no matter the differences each felt with the news of Joan's death, each and every one of them had the same sentiment about my mom's life. Joan was special. I heard about the joy and laughter she had brought to their lives. I heard about the invaluable gift of friendship my mom both imparted and accepted from these remarkable girlfriends. Although the task was overwhelming and heartbreaking, to listen to these women tell me about the Joan they knew was perfectly beautiful. I'll cherish their words forever.

Thursday, the ninth of August was a day to spend with Steve. We had plenty to do. My mother taught me to be a list maker and cross off each completed task with enthusiasm. The first order of the day was sobbing. It wasn't on the list; it came when it wanted. We went to the mall. Steve had a tux fitting for Bonnie's wedding. I wanted to look at dresses for the funeral. I had spent some time recently at the mall looking for a mother of the bride dress, and now I needed a daughter of the dead dress. I couldn't find anything I thought was appropriate. We went out for lunch. We drove to Mom's apartment to begin the process of packing and moving. We took one load away. We drove to Lee's place to fix something wrong on his car. We went to the local food warehouse to buy things to eat and drink. We knew company was coming. We went home and straightened up the house for company. I called Fran. I called a friend from our old neighborhood. Both knew Joan well and promised to pass the word to anyone they thought should know. I called a coworker who also promised to share with those who needed to know. I thought about how lame it was that my father hadn't called me to tell me he's sorry I lost my mother. That hurt. Steve and I made a few drinks, surprised by all our accomplishments that day, and went to bed without supper.

Friday, the tenth of August was just as busy. Lee needed shoes. I needed hose. I decided to wear a classy dress of Joan's to her service. It fit me beautifully. She knew how to buy a nice dress. We removed another load from her apartment. I gathered pictures together to place in the church for the service. We had a three o'clock rehearsal appointment at the church. I was unaware that funerals or memorial services had rehearsals. On my way to the car, preparing to go to the church, I noticed a newspaper in the driveway. With all the running around and preparing for the next day's events, I forgot about buying a newspaper. Friday's paper was going to run the obituary that Scott wrote, and that newspaper lying in my driveway reminded me of the one chore I forgot about that day. The words "complimentary paper" were written on the outside covering. I had never before received a complimentary paper delivered to my door. To receive one on this day had to have been a gift from Joan. Awesome. I looked up to the sky to thank her, and I laughed. I opened the paper and looked down to read her obituary, and I cried. I could hear her talking to me. "Candy, there you are running around making sure everything is just right. You have company coming, and you are feeding everyone. You are making sure your house is clean. You work so hard at everything you do, and it shows. You are amazing. I knew you'd be angry at yourself if you forgot to get the paper today, so I did what I could." I could really hear her. That's just what she'd say. She was good at letting me know how proud she was of my abilities and accomplishments. Her gift to me was so fitting.

We drove to the church. Debbie, Julia and Jayne were on their way from Raleigh. They were meeting us at the church. Debbie was going to sing with Mark during the service. Sound checks, floral arrangement placements, photograph placements, program proofreading, and experiencing what it feels like to be in a pulpit was the extent of the rehearsal.

Later, everyone went back to our home, like Mom knew we would. I didn't mind; I enjoyed having people over to my house. Debbie and the girls were staying with us. I was so glad we remained close with Mark's first wife and his children. Bonnie and Joe arrived. We made a big circle of lawn chairs in the empty basement and listened to Mark play the guitar. We sang along to "Mr. Bojangles," "House of the Rising Sun," and of course, "You Are My Sunshine." We drank beer and wine. We laughed and cried. We ordered Chinese food for dinner.

We felt prepared for Saturday, the day we were to celebrate the life of our mother, Joan.

Chapter 16 The Funeral

Mom, you would have loved the funeral. It was beautiful. The day was sunny, and your church was full of those you loved. Your family was present. Your girlfriends were there. People who worked with Scott and people who worked with me attended. Your old neighbors came. Lea Anne and Phil were present. Fran and her sister were there. Your church friends attended. My old neighbors came. Dad and Doris made it. All of these people gathered to celebrate you.

Your Reverend began with a greeting, words of assurance, and a prayer. The congregation sang "Amazing Grace." The Reverend read from the scripture, Psalms 23 and selected verses of 139. She read Philippians 4:8. She then told some personal stories about you. She spoke of your love of the children you interacted with at church. She praised your questioning mind in bible class. She disclosed some stories that came from her notes taken on Wednesday when we were all together talking about you and your amazing spirit. Then, she turned it over to your children. One by one, we rose to share with the congregation our love for you. After all, Mom, you taught me to never be afraid of standing up and being heard.

Scott and Diana walked to the pulpit. Scott reminded everyone about your famous sense of humor. He honored your quick wit and reminded everyone that your ability to joke and be silly was one of the last pieces to leave your lovable personality. Diana read a poem she wrote describing the gentle and generous Joan. They stepped down, and I stepped up.

Mom, I looked out at all the faces of family and friends staring at me. Their expressions of pure empathy made speaking easy. I started with the line, "My mother treated strangers like friends, and she treated friends like family." My voice cracked once, and I felt the Reverend's hand touch my back. After a short pause, I was able to describe your unbelievable kindness with ease. I told the congregation about the way you treated strangers. From bank customers to people you met out in the community, you always modeled respectful behavior. You would strike up a conversation with everyone you met, and you made each person who crossed your path feel special. I told them how you would make funny faces at the kids to make them laugh while they waited in line with their parents for a bank teller to be open. I told the congregation about the way you treated my friends. You always made them feel welcome in the house, and you always had a kind thing to say. My friends remembered. I told them how much I loved and appreciated hearing, "Your mom is so nice," while growing up. You made me proud. I told the congregation about your kindness directed toward your grandchildren. You gave them fond memories at Grandma's house. You would bring down boxes of old clothes from the attic, and the kids would play dress up. I told them about all the drawing and artistic creating that took place with Grandma. You went through these rituals with all of your grandchildren, and when they were all at Grandma's together, the fun multiplied. You were a grandma who never scolded, a grandma who laughed a lot. Ideal.

I read a beautiful poem I found in my book of life prayers from around the world. It reminded me of you, Mom. Then, as I was leaving the altar, I told everyone that I was wearing your dress. I don't know why. When I put the dress on that morning with my hair still up in a towel and no makeup on my face, funny, I looked like you. You were looking at me from the mirror.

Mark climbed the steps to the altar next. He spoke about your appreciation of the arts. He honored your belief that museum trips and music in the house was an integral part of raising children. He even mentioned your love of puns and the written word. He thought you might like to know that "funeral" is an anagram that can be rearranged to read "real fun." He read an email that he had received from a childhood friend the day before. This friend described his memories of Joan, the All American Mom, who let the boys jam in the basement. Then we sang the song.

"You Are My Sunshine" by now had become your theme song. Mark and Debbie sang the verses in perfect harmony. Mark asked the congregation to join in the chorus. " You are my sunshine, my only sunshine/ You make me happy when skies are gray/You'll never know dear, how much I love you/Please, don't take my sunshine away" The tears fell for you, Mom.

The reverend asked the congregation if anyone would like to come up to the pulpit and say a few words about you. Diana's oldest son rose. He movingly told everyone that he was the recipient of all the beautiful character traits so eloquently described by your children. He told them about the first time he met you. He was ten and lived with his mom and Scott. You had traveled out to California to visit. He said how meaningful it was to him when you told him to call you Grandma. He told everyone that these past few years, when we would all get together and you would repeat your favorite jokes, we would all join in, not with annoyance over hearing them for the umpteenth time, but because it was so joyous to finish the punch line all together, laughing all the way. He sat back down, and a man I had never seen before, a member of your church, stood up and told everyone that you were one gracious lady. You touched people, Mom.

Mark played the guitar and sang one more song. The reverend closed with a prayer and a benediction. We all convened in the Fellowship Hall to greet the people who took time out of their day to pay tribute to you, Mom. Churches provide good work in time of death.

I thanked my friends and coworkers for coming. I smiled and shook hands and enjoyed stories by your friends and coworkers. Bonnie and Lee smiled and shook hands as they met many of your acquaintances for the first time. Those acquaintances sure knew about your family, however. You bragged a lot it seems. The clan of Joan moved to our home for the last time to continue fellowship in your honor. Scott and Diana, their kids and grandkids, Mark and his girlfriend, Debbie and the girls, Steve and I, and our kids all enjoyed a feeling of contentment and closure together.

At one point during the afternoon, I walked upstairs and found Lee in the guestroom staring at a picture on the wall. It was the Lion King watercolor you painted for Lee's room when he was a little boy. At the bottom you wrote, "The Lion King for Lee by Grandma." Lee was crying.

The subdued afternoon wore down. The satisfaction of a successful memorial helped to begin the official healing process. Everyone left the house right before the sun went down. I went to bed right after the sun went down. Before I closed my eyes, I made myself a promise that I would continue to live what you taught me and to teach others about your ways, Mom.

Scott called me Sunday morning to let me know of the gift you gave to him. Steve and I were sitting on the deck enjoying a cup of coffee when the phone rang. Scott told me that as he was walking down his driveway to pick up his Sunday paper, he noticed one single white flower blooming among the reds and purples he had planted that spring in his mailbox garden. A white flower had never appeared there before. That was brilliant, Mom. Scott, your peacemaking son, looked up and smiled with gratitude upon discovering the flower. He felt it was a thank you for the service, a sign that all was well. Your final gifts to each of your children were just right Mom. You knew us well.

I hung up the phone and returned to Steve who was taking in the beauty of the morning sun as it filtered through the trees producing those special, long morning shadows we both loved so much. I scanned the yard full of flowers, shrubs, bird feeders, a birdbath, and so very much green lingering from the back woods. I smiled at our beloved brick work. That patio Steve and I created and labored over is a perfect metaphor for life, isn't it Mom? We should all strive for a level surface before laying a foundation. We should put down foundation material that is strong and supportive, yet flexible enough to allow for unplanned movement. The bricks represent the lessons, the people, and the events we all experience in life. We should examine each brick closely to expose the most beautiful side and place that positive side upward. Each brick connects to the next, relying on one another for stability and boundaries. Sometimes, wayward roots emerge from below the surface causing a brick to jut up out of line. Skilled hands must sever and discard the root before replacing the brick. Sometimes, heavy rains fall from above the surface causing a brick to sink down out of line. Skilled hands must add to the washed away foundation before replacing the brick. But most of the time, the patio gets what it needs to stay intact. Sunny days warm and bond the bricks allowing them to age comfortably. Nature finds the warmth irresistible. Family and friends gather on the bricks, their weight compressing the foundation to promote a long lasting durability. Laughter ricochets off the surface back into the people. With craftsmanship and nurturing, the patio can last forever.

Mom, I'm grateful we took the time to walk together on many brick patios before you left this world. And Mom, I hope you know that I will always remember you as my sunshine.

ABOUT THE AUTHOR

Candace lives in the suburbs of Atlanta with her husband and the family dog and cat. She works in public education as a counselor. She enjoys spending time with her family and friends. She misses her mom.

Contact her at:
candaceminorcomstock@gmail.com

Made in the USA
Lexington, KY
27 August 2012